PRAISE FОɌ

Yoga for Times of Change

"Written in an accessible, personal, intelligent, honest, informed, and encouraging manner, *Yoga for Times of Change* gives readers authentic, deeply yogic ways to move through difficult yet inevitable times of change in their lives."

—William K. Mahony, PhD,
professor of Religious Studies, Davidson College

"Written in the soothing voice of a calm, strong, and compassionate yoga teacher, Nina Zolotow draws wisdom from ancient yoga texts, knowledge from Western psychology and neuroscience, and understanding from her own journey through disturbed mind toward balance. *Yoga for Times of Change* is a wise and honest book that offers us profound insight and safe practice. It's a treasured addition to my library!"

—Amy Weintraub,
author of *Yoga for Depression*

"*Yoga for Times of Change* is a wonderfully heartfelt and authentic book offering a rich collection of techniques to help us navigate the ups and downs of this thing called LIFE. Whether you are looking for ways to cope with stress, anger, anxiety, or depression, this book contains a wealth of profound yogic tools for transformation. Best of all, they are presented in a way that makes them easily accessible even for those without any previous yoga experience."

—Eva Norlyk Smith,
PhD, C-RYT, founder and president of YogaUOnline

Yoga for Times of Change

Practices and Meditations for
Moving Through Stress, Anxiety, Grief,
and Life's Transitions

NINA ZOLOTOW

SHAMBHALA

Shambhala Publications, Inc.
2129 13th Street
Boulder, Colorado 80302
www.shambhala.com

Cover art: Apola/iStock
Cover design: Laura Shaw
Interior design: Kate Huber-Parker

9 8 7 6 5 4 3 2 1

First Edition
Printed in the United States of America

Shambhala Publications makes every effort to print on acid-free, recycled paper.
Shambhala Publications is distributed worldwide by
Penguin Random House, Inc., and its subsidiaries.

Library of Congress Cataloging-in-Publication Data
Names: Zolotow, Nina, author.
Title: Yoga for times of change: practices and meditations for moving through stress, anxiety, grief, and life's transitions / Nina Zolotow.
Description: Boulder, Colorado: Shambhala, 2022.
Identifiers: LCCN 2021049124 | ISBN 9781611809282 (trade paperback)
Subjects: LCSH: Yoga—Therapeutic use. | Mental illness—Alternative treatment.
Classification: LCC RM727.Y64 Z65 2022 | DDC 613.7/046—dc23/eng/202111102
LC record available at https://lccn.loc.gov/2021049124

To the memory of Donald Moyer,

who taught me and inspired me

in more ways than I can say

CONTENTS

PREFACE   ix

USING THIS BOOK   xiii

1   Introduction   1

2   Coping with Change   15

3   Stress Management for When You're Stressed   65

4   Moving Through Anger, Anxiety, and Depression   85

5   Moving Through Grief   143

6   Adapting to Physical Changes   169

7   Being Present   187

8   Making Peace with Change   223

ACKNOWLEDGMENTS   261

APPENDIX: TIPS FOR STAYING SAFE   265

NOTES   269

INDEX   275

PREFACE

Dearly beloved
We are gathered here today
To get through this thing called life
—Prince Rogers Nelson, from "Let's Go Crazy"

After weeks of oppressive gray clouds and unending drizzle, Cambridge, England, was beautiful that summer day. The sky was a glorious blue, Midsummer Common was a glorious green, and the tidy flowerbeds were in full bloom. My one-year-old daughter was bouncing up and down in her British pushchair, smiling and laughing as she pointed a chubby finger at the baby ducks and the family of swans that were swimming slowly down the River Cam. I, on the other hand, had tears streaming down my face and didn't care who saw me crying in public. I'd had another sleepless night, and no matter what I did—going for a run when my husband got home, hiring a sitter so I could go to a weekly yoga class, taking a break with a night out with my new Canadian friends—my insomnia was relentless and my weight was continuing to drop.

Moving to England when I was five months pregnant had been hard for me. I'd left behind a full-time job as a technical writer and documentation manager and a circle of friends in Boston for life as a "resident alien housewife" in a picturesque but very provincial university town where I knew not a single person and where everyone I met, whether through the university or in the town, saw me only as a "young mum." But recently my situation had become even more challenging because my husband, Brad, was looking for a permanent job and was talking about moving somewhere else new— again—and to places where I had no wish to live—instead of returning to California, where we'd both grown up. I felt trapped because while I didn't want to split up our family, I also didn't want to move somewhere else where I felt like I didn't belong. Then my father had a life-changing stroke, and my parents, who had been living for the last year in London, moved back to Los Angeles to figure out what was next for them. That's when the insomnia started.

When I finally went to see my family doctor, as my daughter sat at our feet playing with my wallet and keys he said, "I'm not surprised." His office was across the street from Cambridge University, so he'd seen the same situation many times—wife of a postdoctoral fellow or graduate student, baby in a foreign country, blah, blah, blah. The bottom line was that I was having a nervous breakdown, and he ultimately diagnosed me with agitated depression.

Thanks to a combination of therapy and medication, I recovered from my breakdown and my marriage survived. But I was left with so many questions: Why had this happened to me? I wasn't against change and uncertainty, so why was I having such a hard time dealing with it now, for the first time? Was there anything I could do to prevent this all from happening again? And who was I now when I had turned out to be much more vulnerable that I had ever imagined?

That was the beginning of my personal journey to understand change—how to adapt to it and how to accept it. I tried more therapy, I read books about emotional illness, I took up swimming, and I studied creative writing. It wasn't until years later that I learned that something I had already been doing for exercise—yoga—held the answers I was looking for. I didn't find those answers, though, by just going to weekly yoga classes. It was only when I started studying yoga in depth, practicing yoga regularly at home, taking special workshops with a variety of teachers, and reading both modern and ancient books on yoga that I learned how I could use yoga to help myself and then later on to help others as well. That's why I'm writing this book now, with the aim of making it as easy as possible for you to learn—all in one place—all the wonderful things I now know about how yoga can help during times of change.

To deepen my understanding of both human nature and why yoga is so powerful for helping us adapt to and accept change, I decided to branch out in my studies, delving into human physiology, brain science, psychology, and even human evolution. I didn't have a curriculum to follow, so I created my own. For a number of years, I read many books and articles, and even consulted directly with various scientific experts. I was fascinated to see that many contemporary scientific discoveries support the original observations about human nature that the ancient yogis made, and this background was very helpful to me in understanding the "why" and the "how" of yoga, along with the "what." So I'm including some of that background here in this book, along with all the information about yoga.

Yes, I'll admit it, this book is jam-packed with both simple, down-to-earth practices and lofty ideas. It's my hope that at least some them will help you, as Prince said, "get through this thing called life."

USING THIS BOOK

This book will describe many ways you can use yoga to balance yourself when you're confronted with the physical, emotional, and mental changes that life brings, and it provides suggestions for how you can become more comfortable with life's ups and downs by learning to live your everyday life in a yogic way. I'm including both ancient and modern techniques: yoga poses of all kinds, breath practices, relaxation, meditation, and yogic tools for working with the mind.

Rather than being a "program," the chapters in this book present a collection of techniques and ideas that I've been gathering for decades. Maybe the most important thing I've learned about using yoga for times of change—or for that matter yoga for any time—is that everyone is different, in their abilities, preferences, and personal approaches to yoga. So, like those one-size-fits-all outfits that never look good on me, there is no one-size-fits-all yoga that works for everyone. That's why instead of "recommending" a single way to practice for times of change, I'm going to provide you with a large variety of suggestions to choose from so you can discover what works best for you. As you read through this book—or jump directly to a chapter that addresses something you're going through—keep in mind that you can try whatever appeals to you. And if that doesn't work, there will be something else you can try.

I'm also taking a somewhat different approach to the way I show yoga poses in this book. Because I wanted to make the poses in this book as accessible as possible, I thought to myself: Who needs the most help—beginners or those who already have experience? People who need to use props to make the poses safe and comfortable, or people who have been practicing for years and can do the classic poses with ease? The answer was obvious. That's why throughout this book, for almost all poses, I'll be showing versions of the classic poses that use props and other techniques to make them more accessible. If you're used to practicing these poses a different way, of course you can practice the versions that you already know and love instead. I'm also including information in chapter 6 to show you how to modify your own poses, so, if for any reason, you need a different version of a pose than the one I show, you can change the pose to suit yourself. And if you'd like to practice any of these sequences along with a video, Barrie Risman has made a series of videos in which she teaches all the sequences in this book, and they are available on her website at https://www.barrierisman.com/yogafortimesofchange.

Finally, it's always a good idea to keep safety in mind as you practice yoga poses. See the appendix for a list of tips for how you can make your home practice—as well as your classroom experiences—as safe as possible.

By the way, many of the quotes in this book are from my blog, *Yoga for Healthy Aging*, which is on the Yoga for Times of Change website. To find all posts I've referenced and hundreds more that might be of interest, go to https://www.yogafortimesof change.com/blog.

IMPORTANT: The information in this book is not intended as a substitute for personalized medical advice. The reader should consult a physician before beginning this or any exercise program. The author and the publisher assume no responsibility for pain or injury experienced from the practice of exercises presented here.

Yoga for Times of Change

1

Introduction

Life is an ever-rolling wheel
And every day is the right one.
—Mumon Gensen

On Wednesday, September 9, 2020, I woke up later than usual because it was still dark outside when it should have been light. Confused, I opened the curtains and saw that the entire sky was a dark-orange color, as if it were night but an orange night instead of dark-blue one. Previously my husband Brad and I had spent many days inside our house, windows closed against unhealthy smoke-filled air from several different fires that ringed the San Francisco Bay Area. But that morning, we learned, a combination of the fog coming in from the Pacific (which brought a blessed relief from the previous days of heat) and a high-level layer of smoke from the fire in the Sierras that settled above the fog had created a barrier that prevented most of the sun's light waves from penetrating down to the earth's surface.

What could we do? We decided to simply go about our day, with me working on my book in my home office and Brad working remotely from his home office downstairs. But this dark-orange sky, which continued for almost the entire day, was deeply unsettling on two levels. First, it was so unexpected. While we know that change is an intrinsic part of nature, that the color of the sky should change so drastically had previously been unimaginable. Everyone was saying it seemed like our city had been transported to another planet! And, second, what did this new development portend? Was every fire season in California going to be this extreme from now on? Were there more dark-orange skies in our future? Should we be thinking of moving somewhere else? Even though we were safe for the time being, it was a long and difficult day for us to get through.

For all of us, times of change include the ordinary ups and downs of life that affect us as individuals—you know, the marshmallows and walnuts in the rocky road ice cream of life. These changes can be physical or emotional, temporary or permanent, minor or major. And they include births and deaths, temporary or chronic health problems, important relationships beginning and ending, moving from one place or job to another, or transitions to a new phase in life.

Times of change also include periods of societal, political, and environmental upheaval or transformation in our communities and across the world. All four of my grandparents were immigrants from Eastern Europe who came to the United States as teenagers, and I often reflect on the long list of changes they experienced throughout their lives. In addition to the personal challenges of moving to a new country where they didn't speak the language, they lived through World War I, the influenza pandemic, the women's suffrage movement, the Great Depression, World War II and the Holocaust (during which my maternal grandmother lost most of her family), the Cold War, the civil rights movement the space age, and more.

And recently, during 2020 and 2021, we all lived through changes in our communities and across the world that affected us as individuals as much as the everyday events in our personal lives did. After all, the pandemic disrupted everyone's lives worldwide, causing loss of life and other hardships, forcing us to change the way we were living and working, and making us put our plans for the future on hold. That year was also a period of extreme weather and social upheaval. We quickly learned how all these types of changes are not only hard to live through but raise unsettling questions about what the future holds

All in all, change and uncertainty are intrinsic aspects of life on earth. The ancient yogis understood this, and in yoga, one of the basic principles of reality is that the material world, which includes your body-mind as well as other beings and external objects, is by its nature ever changing. As T. K. V. Desikachar says in *The Heart of Yoga*:

Although in yoga everything we see and experience is true and real, all form and all content are in a constant state of flux. This concept of continual change is known as *parinamavada*.[1]

The ancient yogis also observed that even though the nature of the material world is that it is impermanent and in a constant state of flux, we humans often suffer when we experience change, loss, and uncertainty. In recent times, scientists who study human evolution have come up with very compelling explanations for *why* change and impermanence cause so much suffering. Basically, evolution wired us to survive and to have as many offspring as possible. So when we face times of change, we experience a variety of painful reactions, such as stress, anger, fear, depression, and grief that will prompt us to find a way to survive the "dangers" we are facing. However, what once helped us to survive during more primitive times may not always serve us in the modern world because not everything our nervous system interprets as "danger" is actually dangerous. For example, we can be terrified of public speaking, full of rage because someone takes our parking space, or humiliated after an interaction with a stranger we will never see again. In addition, many of us long to experience more peace, contentment, and happiness rather than being buffeted about by painful reactions to so many things in our environments.

Fortunately, as we evolved to survive, we also evolved to be curious about the universe and capable of self-awareness. This means that we have the ability to observe our own reactions to what we experience, which can lead us to a deeper understanding of human nature and what causes us to experience suffering. The ancient yogis did exactly this. They systematically identified the causes of human suffering, and from there they came up with many different ways to reduce that suffering and even to liberate us from it completely. The Bhagavad Gita defines a yogi as one

Who unperturbed by changing conditions sits apart and watches and says "the powers of nature go round," and remains firm and shakes not. (14.23)[2]

To learn how to use yoga to stay calm, steady, and content during times of change, it's very helpful to start with a basic understanding of why our human nature makes living through times of change particularly challenging. So before you dive into the suggestions for ways of using yoga to help you cope during challenging times in chapters 2 through 8, here's some background about human nature and about yoga itself to provide you with a basic foundation for making decisions about which yoga practices can help you adapt to and accept whatever changes you're going through.

Understanding Human Nature:
Attraction and Aversion

One of our most basic features as human animals is having very strong feelings about what is good for us and what is dangerous or should be avoided. And, as is true for all animals, these strong reactions to what we encounter in our environment help us to stay alive. In his book *Why Buddhism Is True*, psychologist Robert Wright says that when feelings first appeared in the living world, "their mission was to take care of the organism, specifically to get it to approach things that are good for it (like food) and avoid things that are bad for it (like toxins)."[3]

Because these strong reactions to what we encounter in our environment are so fundamental to our nature, we now experience the same strong feelings we have about the basics of food, sex, and shelter for things we encounter in modern times, whether serious, such as feeling terrible anxiety about layoffs at work or anger over a news story about the plight of people halfway across the word from you, or frivolous, such as having a crush on a celebrity you've never even met or feeling angry at someone who took the last pint of your favorite ice cream before you could grab it.

And whenever we encounter anything, whether basic or modern, that we feel is beneficial for us, we become attached to it. That's because evolution wired us to want to repeat experiences that cause us pleasure. Otherwise, we'd eat or have sex just once and be satisfied forever, which would certainly prevent us from surviving long enough to have children. So, to ensure our own survival and that of our offspring—which is how our genes stay in the gene pool—we evolved to keep wanting the things we feel we need for our well-being and happiness.

Getting what we desire makes us temporarily happy, but then that happiness wears off and we yearn to repeat the experience. And being completely unable to get the things we're attached to, well, that really makes us suffer. I remember all too well watching toddlers crying and fighting over a toy they desperately wanted. Even as adults, we all experience that kind of heartbreak, whether over the end of an important relationship, losing family heirlooms in a robbery, or seeing your community destroyed by a natural disaster.

Ancient yogis identified attachment to pleasure (*raga*) as one of the causes of suffering. In Patanjali's Yoga Sutras pleasure is included as the third in a list of five "afflictions" in sutra II.3:

> The five afflictions which disturb the equilibrium of consciousness are: ignorance or lack of wisdom, ego, pride of the ego or the sense of "I," attachment to pleasure, aversion to pain, fear of death and clinging to life.[4]

In his *Yoga Sutras of Patanjali* Edwin Bryant explains attachment to pleasure this way:

> One who has experienced pleasure in the past recollects it and hankers to repeat the experience in the present or future, or to attain the means of repeating the experience; it is dwelling on past experiences that constitutes attachment.[5]

With change, there is always loss. Some change is just a loss, whether the death of a loved one, loss of your job or home, or the end of an important relationship. And losing the things that we feel we need for our well-being and survival causes suffering in the form of stressful emotions such as frustration, anger, depression, fear, anxiety, and grief. During the pandemic, I knew a number of people who cried every day because their grief over our worldwide losses was so intense.

But all change involves some kind of loss, even when it's a basically a positive change. For example, moving to a new place or changing jobs may mean leaving people you care about behind. Having a baby—especially your first one—typically means changing your way of life and giving up many activities you were attached to. So, even for positive changes, there is usually some discomfort. I remember being so nervous the day I was married even though we just did a casual city-hall thing and were already living together.

On the other hand, because we evolved to be repelled by things that aren't beneficial for us, having to do things that we dislike or that make us uncomfortable or afraid also causes suffering. For example, for a few years my young niece used to panic whenever it was time to wash her hair because she was so afraid to get her head wet. Even as adults, we all feel that same kind of resistance, whether to taking a major exam, having to resolve a serious conflict with a neighbor, or going to the dentist.

Ancient yogis identified aversion to pain (*dvesa*) as one of the causes of suffering. In sutra II.3 from the Yoga Sutras quoted earlier it is fourth in a list of five "afflictions." Edwin Bryant explains aversion this way:

> Aversion, *dvesa*, after all, is the flip side of the same coin as attachment. When we resist or resent something, or are angry or frustrated over something, it is because of a remembrance that this thing has caused us pain in the past.[6]

Some changes mean that we will need to do things that we're afraid of or that we dislike. Divorce might entail, for example, sharing custody of children and splitting up your possessions, and for some just the thought of living alone can be frightening or depressing. The pandemic, of course, brought a whole host of changes we all disliked, from not being able to visit friends and loved ones to having to wait in line at the market. But even ordinary changes can mean doing things we're averse to—I mean, who likes packing up their house to move?

All in all, attachment and aversion create very basic and strong emotions in human beings that challenge our equanimity and sense of contentment when we experience any kind of change. With this understanding, you can start to question your attachments to the way life used to be and your aversions to some of the effects that change brings.

Counting on the Future

Be in peace in pleasure and pain, in gain and in loss, in victory or in the loss of a battle. (2.38)
—*Bhagavad Gita*, trans. Juan Mascaro

Another basic characteristic we have as human animals that affects our experience of change is the urge to plan for the future. This basic impulse is triggered by our memories of past failures and successes as well as our expectations about times to come.

All organisms capable of long-term memory are necessarily oriented toward the future. A feature of memory apparently unique to humans, however, is the degree to which the decisions and plans that we make are based on representations that are future oriented—imaginings of specific events located forward in time.[7]

Our ability to plan for the future is one of the qualities that made us so successful as a species. During the hunter-gatherer era, concern about the future helped us stockpile food for the winter and eventually led to the development of agriculture. And we also made plans to avoid repeating dangerous mistakes, for example, by organizing a hunting party to take down a large animal instead of hunting solo. In fact, this ability to plan for the future is said to be the basis for most—if not all of—modern civilization, including the development of writing and our various systems of laws and forms of government. And all this planning for the future allowed us to stay alive long enough to have offspring, who themselves stayed alive long enough to produce their own offspring, and so on.

The powerful urge to plan is as beneficial to us for our survival in the modern world as it was in more primitive times. For example, we benefit from stocking up on supplies and boarding up windows in advance of a big storm and from saving money for retirement. Our urge to make plans for the future does tend to be associated with stressful emotions, however. Of course, anxiety, fear, and anger in the present motivate us to make plans for the future. But also memories of our past experiences, especially painful ones, such as shame, guilt, regret, anger, and grief, teach us not to make the same mistakes and to take steps to create a future with potentially different outcomes. Then because planning is so important to us, we become very attached to the plans we make and to the outcomes we're hoping for.

But, as you know, many of our plans don't work out because circumstances that our plans depend on can change. When that happens, because of our attachment to our plans, if we have to revise the way see our future, we can experience very stressful emotions. For example, before the United Kingdom voted to leave the European Union, many EU citizens who were living and working in the United Kingdom—and who thought of the country where they were living as their home—had plans for the future that depended on them staying in the United Kingdom. But, after Brexit was enacted, many of these people had to move to different countries, where they needed to search for new jobs, find new homes, and start their lives all over again, all of which are major stressors.

Sometimes changes make things so uncertain that we can't even make plans! Then because we're so oriented toward the future, living without plans—being in a state of uncertainty—is uncomfortable for us. All we can do is wait to see how things play out, and waiting isn't anyone's idea of fun. Right now, like a lot of people, I can't yet make actual plans to see close family members who live far away, but I often find myself fantasizing anyway in ridiculous detail about what I'll do when I do see them.

In addition, our orientation toward the future may even cause us to overlook what's happening in the present. For example, I knew someone who was so focused on the milestones they had mapped out for the future—the list was literally on the refrigerator—that they failed to see how unhappy they were making their partner until it was too late.

So both our basic urge to make plans and our feelings of attachment to the plans we make need to be balanced with an understanding that the future is always uncertain. From there, you can start to accept that even when you make carefully thought-out plans, things often don't turn out as you hope. Then you're ready to use your yoga practice in new ways to become more comfortable with the ever-changing nature of reality and the uncertainty that your future holds.

Yoga and Change

For the pleasures that come from the world bear in them sorrows to come. They come and they go, they are transient: not in them do the wise find joy.

But he who on this earth, before his departure, can endure the storms of desire and wrath, this man is a Yogi, this man has joy.

He has inner joy, he has inner gladness, and he has found inner Light. (5.22–24)
—*Bhagavad Gita*, trans. Juan Mascaro

Developed in India, yoga is an evolving body of spiritual values and techniques—both ancient and modern—intended to "liberate" practitioners from the suffering caused by life in an ever-changing material world. The yoga tradition includes many widely differing paths to achieve this state of liberation or permanent "enlightenment." But in all these paths achieving liberation is a long and arduous process, attainable only to those who are very committed and willing to make many sacrifices, with the possible exception of a very few people who experience an instantaneous awakening. You can think of this goal of liberation as the very peak of the yoga mountain, a peak that only a very few will reach.

I realized many years ago that even though yoga was so helpful to me for adapting to and accepting change in the real world, I wasn't going to even attempt to reach yoga's highest peak. Instead, I set my sights on an important way station on the path to yoga's highest peak: equanimity. Although equanimity in everyday life wasn't the ultimate goal of traditional yoga, the ancient yogis understood that focusing on your spiritual practice isn't really feasible if you are constantly being buffeted about by intense emotions or your personal life is in complete disarray. So they came up with many different practices to help you stay steady and calm during ever-changing circumstances, and to be more content with what you have and what you don't have. These practices run the whole gamut from yoga's ethical guidelines and the asana practice to breath practices, concentration, meditation, and yogic tools for working with your thoughts.

Although there is a very wide range of definitions for exactly what yoga is, the Bhagavad Gita, an early yoga text and one of the most popular of all time, actually uses the term "equanimity" in stanza 2.48: "Yoga is called equanimity."[8] The original Sanskrit word here, which Georg Feuerstein translates as equanimity, is *samatva*. Feuerstein explains the meaning of *samatva* in this context: "The Sanskrit word *samatva* means literally 'sameness' or 'evenness' and has all kinds of overtones, including 'balance' and 'harmony.' Essentially it is an attitude of looking dispassionately at life and being unruffled by its ups and downs."[9] I like this particular definition because it reflects my personal experience with yoga. As my longtime friend and yoga buddy Melitta Rorty always says, "We practice yoga because it makes our lives better." And while "sameness" and "evenness" might not sound that exciting, the Bhagavad Gita in the quote above tells us that cultivating equanimity ultimately leads to "inner joy" and "inner gladness."

The thing is, it's important for us all to recognize that yoga comes from India and that it originally developed there as a spiritual practice, not as a fitness system or wellness program. But just as when you take a walk in nature and find delights and surprises around every bend in the trail, you don't have to climb the whole yoga mountain to find gems of wisdom that will help you in your everyday life. So if achieving a state of complete equanimity, or "being unruffled" by life's ups and downs, feels like an impossible goal, you can just head toward the equanimity way station at your own speed. As the Bhagavad Gita says: "No step is lost on this path, and no dangers are found. And even a little progress is freedom from fear" (2.40).[10]

In *Why Buddhism Is True*, Robert Wright says something similar about why he practices mindfulness meditation: "The object of the game isn't to reach Liberation and Enlightenment—with a capital L and E—on some distant day, but rather to become a bit more liberated and a bit more enlightened on a not-so-distant day."[11] "A bit more enlightened" sounds like an excellent goal to me!

Although I've been quoting primarily from the Bhagavad Gita in this section, the yoga paths described in that text are not the only ones that can help you cultivate equanimity, be more content with what you have and what you don't have, and lead you to "inner joy." In chapter 8, I'll provide some basic information about some of these paths and how they differ from each other. But whatever their differences, all types of yoga recognize the existence of suffering due to ever-changing circumstances in the material world, and all provide ways to alleviate that suffering. And in all paths, important positive side effects of alleviating your personal suffering and learning to be more content with what you have and what you don't have are that you'll also cause less suffering for others and be a better citizen of the world.

This is why over the years I've found it helpful to open my mind to a variety of yoga paths and why this book presents techniques and ideas I've gleaned from many different teachers and yoga texts. In *The Yoga Sutras of Patanjali*, Bryant refers to combining elements from different yoga paths as "a kind of *kitchorie* Yoga" (*kitchorie* being a traditional Indian dish of rice, legumes, spices, and other ingredients, the recipe for which varies not only from region to region but from cook to cook).[12] He says that this approach is not only "understandable" but is perhaps "inevitable," because the same type of approach occurred within the Indic culture itself throughout its own history. However, because I want to prevent confusion about which practices are ancient and which are modern as well as about what came from which yoga text, as I discuss various techniques and concepts, I'll let you know where they come from.

How Yoga Helps in Times of Change

Yoga has helped me through everything—divorce, widowhood, financial disaster, and so on. I never thought about it like that because I've practiced yoga (not just asana) for over fifty years so it's like breathing.

—Beth Gibbs, yoga therapist and author

During the afternoon of what I'm now calling the Dark-Orange Sky Day, I practiced yoga. I meditated and practiced a stress-management pose to help me maintain my equanimity. And because I couldn't take a walk that day, I also practiced active yoga poses for exercise, to release physical stress, and to help lift my spirits a bit. In this way, I was using my yoga practice to adapt to changes I was experiencing that very strange day and also to accept the new reality that I was facing. At the same time my friend Bob, who lives a few blocks away, turned to yoga breath practices (pranayama) to relieve his feelings of anxiety. He chose breath practices because he has learned that in general pranayama helps him to "regulate acute moods."

Yoga is especially powerful for helping you adapt to changes because it includes both ancient and modern techniques that enable you to move back into balance when you're experiencing challenges and to fortify yourself for the future. And the large number of options allows you to choose the poses and practices that work best for you, for your particular needs and in your particular situation.

Here are the main ways that yoga can help you move back into balance when changes big or small are throwing you off:

- Choosing yoga poses to balance you. Various yoga poses can affect your moods, stress levels, and energy levels in different ways. When you're experiencing feelings of stress, anger, anxiety, depression, or grief, you can choose poses to relax you, uplift you, quiet you, stimulate you, or release your pent-up energy or emotion. And the poses themselves can easily be adapted to your current physical abilities and energy levels.
- Selecting breath practices to balance you. Yoga's breath practices provide you with a key to your nervous system, allowing you to calm yourself, balance yourself, or stimulate yourself when you want to stabilize yourself during times of change. That in turn can help you regulate your moods.

- **Meditating to quiet your mind.** Yoga's concentration style of meditation provides you with the ability to quiet your mind as well as to reduce your stress levels. The deep peace you experience during practice can be a refuge that you can rely on during times of change.
- **Using yoga's guiding principles to help you make skillful decisions.** The *yamas*, yoga's ethical guidelines for conducting yourself in all your relationships, within your community, and with the world at large, are all intended to help you live with greater equanimity and can guide you in making decisions that will reduce your own suffering as well as that of others.

As important as it is to adapt to change, learning to accept change is essential for staying calm and steady through the ups and downs of life. People who refuse to accept that change is an intrinsic part of life will always suffer because when what they were hoping for doesn't happen or when they find they can no longer do things the way they used to, they may end up "fighting" against their new reality instead of adapting to it. I think we all saw examples of that throughout the pandemic and after the 2020 U.S. election. But when you make peace with change, you not only experience greater contentment, you're also be able to pivot as needed to accommodate whatever your future holds.

Here are the main ways that yoga can help you learn to be content with whatever is arising and to move through times of change with more equanimity and contentment:

- **Practicing yoga poses mindfully.** Practicing yoga poses with awareness— and without judgment—teaches you to listen to what's going on with you mentally, emotionally, and physically on any given day and to let go of attachments to what you think you *should* be experiencing.
- **Using breath practices and meditation to be present.** Both of these train you to be present as you practice, a skill you can then bring into your everyday life. During times of change, being present helps you respond skillfully to what is happening in the moment rather than focusing on what you've lost or panicking about the future.
- **Meditating to learn about your thought patterns.** Observing your thought patterns during meditation can teach you about your automatic reactions to changes both big and small and help you to learn about which of

your thoughts are actually untrue or are not serving you. During times of change, this understanding can help you to let go of habitual thoughts that cause you suffering and to adopt new points of view that foster more contentment.

- Meditating to foster positive emotions. Focusing on cultivating a particular feeling in your meditation, such as compassion, gratitude, joy, forgiveness, or relaxation, can train your mind and heart to respond with those feelings more often in your daily life. This not only increases your personal happiness, but also improves your relationships and encourages you to take actions to help others.
- Using yogic tools to work with your thoughts and emotions. Yoga provides tools to allow you to listen to your emotions and thoughts and to respond skillfully to them. Responding skillfully can include taking actions to help yourself or others or using yogic tools to let go of thoughts and emotions that aren't serving you. This can help you navigate more adeptly through life's transitions and times of change.
- Studying yoga philosophy. Learning about yoga philosophy provides you with alternative ways of thinking about your life, enabling you to be more content with what you have and what you don't have, and to become more comfortable with change. This in turn can make you a better citizen of the world.

I will be covering all these topics—and more—in this book.

2

Coping with Change

A friend of mine confessed to me that when she started sheltering in place during the pandemic, she consoled herself by eating croissants every morning from her local artisan bakery. But she was starting to think that maybe this wasn't such a good idea. What do you typically do when you're going through difficult times? Do you use alcohol, drugs, food, shopping, television, or social media to distract you from thinking or to numb the pain? Do you lash out in irritation or even anger at others or fall into a slump and retreat from them? Or, do you turn to others for sympathy and/or assistance, take a walk, write about your experiences, make art or music, or practice yoga?

We all have coping strategies to help us deal with the disruptions in our lives during times of change. A good coping strategy can help you adjust to a stressful situation and enable you to stay balanced and steady as you navigate through the challenges you are facing. Not all coping strategies are healthy or helpful, however. So it's good to start by taking an honest look at what coping strategies you use that are not really serving you. You can then intentionally substitute a healthier one such as yoga.

Along with turning to my husband and close friends for comfort, my most important coping strategy for many years has been yoga. In fact, the main reason I'm still so committed to yoga after all these years is that it provides me with range of techniques for dealing with all kinds of difficulty.

Rather than just distracting you or numbing you, yoga allows you to self-regulate, which means you can consciously manage your stress levels, moods, and emotions.

When you notice you are stressed out, you can calm yourself. When you are worried or anxious, you can comfort yourself. When you're feeling blue, you can lighten up your mood. And when you're angry, you can cool yourself down.

Now, you may be wondering, when it comes to using yoga as a healthy coping strategy, does it matter which type of yoga you do? The answer is yes. The type of yoga you should practice depends both on how you're feeling at a given time and on what works for you as an individual. That's why I am providing many different choices in this chapter so you can pick the coping skills that are best for you.

1. Centering Yourself with Breath Awareness
2. Calming Yourself with Supported Inverted Poses
3. Resting Your Body and Mind with Savasana
4. Comforting Yourself with Restorative Yoga
5. Taking a Break with a Mindful Asana Practice
6. Releasing Physical Tension by Stretching
7. Improving Your Sleep

Many of the yoga techniques in this chapter enable you to trigger your relaxation response, which is how your body normally responds to safe circumstances or a secure environment. When you trigger the relaxation response, your heart and breath rate slow, your blood pressure drops, your energy usage slows, your digestion and immune systems work more effectively, and your stress-hormone levels gradually decrease. This allows your body and mind to rest, recover, and acquire new energy in a state called "rest and digest." It's a good state to be in! See chapter 3 for more information about your nervous system and how you can use yoga to reduce your stress levels.

Although the general solutions in this chapter may provide you with relief, for those of you who are experiencing major stress, anxiety, mild depression, anger, or grief a targeted approach might be more helpful. So, I'm providing suggestions for ways to address those specific emotions in chapters 4 and 5.

For all the suggestions in this chapter, remember that if something is not working for you, it's not working for you. See When Relaxing Isn't Relaxing for alternatives. And if there are poses in the chapter you can't do for whatever reason, check chapter 6 for ways to adapt the poses for your particular body.

Coping Skill 1: Centering Yourself with Breath Awareness

If you've just been though an intense experience—or maybe even if you're still in the middle one—one of the simplest things you can do to steady yourself is to practice breath awareness. Breath awareness is also a good practice to do on a regular basis when you're going through a period of ongoing stress.

Bringing your awareness to your breath takes you out of your head. It moves your focus from the thoughts racing through your mind—including worries about the future and regrets about the past—to your body and to the present moment. Even a minute or two of practice can help center you or prevent a spike in your stress levels, allowing you to better assess what's happening in the here and now.

For those who aren't already familiar with it, breath awareness means simply observing your natural breath without changing it. With breath awareness, you just watch each breath you take in the here and now, a practice that is both very effective and completely safe.

You can practice breath awareness in a formal way, going to a special place and taking a special position, but you can also just simply stop wherever you are and focus on your breath. You can practice for a long session or even just for a minute or two.

WHEN AND WHERE TO PRACTICE BREATH AWARENESS

Breath awareness is a practice that you can do whenever you want—morning, noon, or night. You can even practice after you go to bed, either before you fall asleep if you want to fall asleep more quickly or sleep more deeply or in the middle of the night if you wake up and can't fall back to sleep.

You can also practice when you're alone or when you're around other people. For example, I have practiced breath awareness in a dental chair while work was being done on me—and received compliments for being such a great patient afterward—as well as during other uncomfortable medical procedures.

If you need a quick fix because something intense is going on or you're just losing patience, whether you're out in public or at home, you can practice breath awareness for twelve breaths or even just for three. For example, my friend Melitta says that she finds practicing for three breaths is really useful for preparing herself for challenging work meetings and for staying patient in long supermarket checkout lines.

And when you need to rest and can't do a seated or standing practice, such as when you are ill or injured, the ability to practice breath awareness is always there for you. The only exceptions might be

- If you're having trouble breathing, whether due to illness or allergies, and focusing on your breath can be frustrating rather than centering.
- If you find focusing on your breath makes you stressed for any reason— some people find it makes them anxious.

In either case, consider using a different focus for your mind, such as a mantra or a visual image (see How to Practice Concentration Meditation on page 208 for ideas). Or, if you have time, try some of the other techniques in this chapter instead.

HOW TO PRACTICE BREATH AWARENESS

You don't need a special place to practice breath awareness. While it's easier to focus on your breath in a quiet environment, you can practice in a busy or noisy place, and you'll still reap the benefits. I even think it's good to practice in a noisy situation intentionally once in a while, so you learn to be comfortable with the idea.

Because you can practice almost anywhere and at any time, you have a large number of options for positions to practice in. For both standing and sitting positions, it's a good idea to adjust your posture so your spine is extended and your head is in line with your spine, as this may allow you to breathe more easily.

Standing. If you're going to be practicing in a public place or just briefly when you're on your own, you can practice breath awareness standing up (a traditional yogic meditation position). If possible, adjust your posture so you stand upright in a nice, symmetrical Mountain pose (Tadasana).

Seated on a chair. If you're going to be practicing in a public place where you are already seated, for example, on an airplane or in a waiting room, or if you are just more comfortable sitting in a chair than on the floor or the floor is not accessible to you, you can practice breath awareness in a comfortable, symmetrical position on your chair.

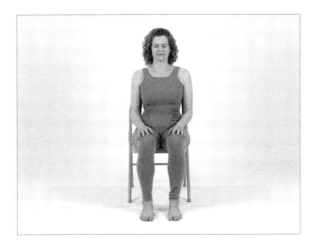

Seated yoga pose. Any stable, comfortable seated yoga pose is good for practicing breath awareness. If you're going to be practicing for more than a couple of minutes, be sure to use appropriate props to ensure you continue to be comfortable. Here are examples of Easy Sitting pose (Sukasana) and Hero pose (Virasana):

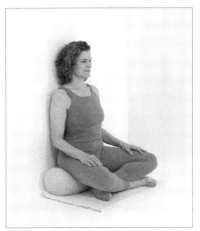

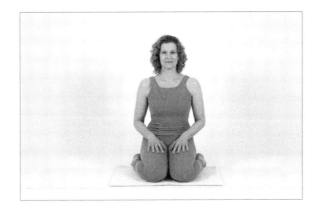

Lying down. You can practice breath awareness lying on a bed or on the floor on a yoga mat, blanket, or carpet. And you have a very large number of choices for positions because in addition to Savasana in all its variations (see Savasana Variations and Alternatives on page 29), you can also practice in any comfortable restorative pose. This includes supine positions, where you're facing up, such as Reclined Cobbler's pose (Supta Baddha Konasana), as well as prone positions, where you're facing the floor, such as Supported Child's pose (Salamba Balasana). If you're feeling anxious, a prone position may be more comforting.

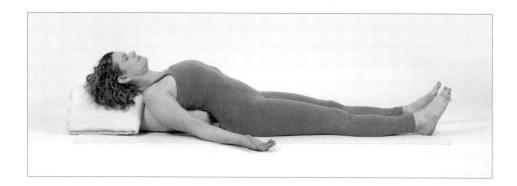

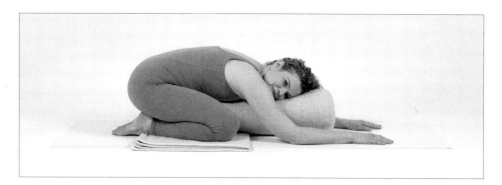

If you practice in an asymmetrical pose, such as a Prone Twist (Supta Bharadvajasana), just make sure to practice on the second side for an equal amount of time. And for all poses, make sure the position is comfortable. If you're lying on your back, using support under your head and under your torso may allow you to breathe more easily (see Savasana Variations and Alternatives on page 29).

For all these positions, you also have the choice of practicing with eyes open or eyes closed. Choose whichever works best for your current circumstances and your personal preference. Both are traditional, in case you wondered. If you do practice with eyes open, try softening your gaze and looking slightly downward, if your circumstances allow it.

How long to practice depends on your circumstances and your goal. A minute of practice or even less can help you center yourself. However, if you want to trigger the relaxation response as I described earlier, you'll need to practice for ten to fifteen minutes in a comfortable seated or reclined position.

TECHNIQUES FOR PRACTICING BREATH AWARENESS

There are many different ways to be "aware" of your breath. However, there are two basic principles to keep in mind. The first is to witness your breath without judgment: Do your best not to judge how well you're breathing. And do your best not judge how well you're paying attention to your breath. When you notice your mind wandering, simply let go of the distracting thoughts and return your focus to your breath.

The second is to refrain from intentionally changing your breath. Allow your inhalations and exhalations to come naturally, and don't try to make them slower, deeper, smoother, and so on. Your breath will naturally change over time as you observe it, especially if you relax as a result of your practice (you need less oxygen when you're relaxed). The point is just to notice the breath.

For those of you who haven't yet learned how to practice breath awareness, here are the four qualities of the breath that Richard Rosen, who is one of my teachers, recommends you observe in his book *The Yoga of Breath*. You can choose any one of the four qualities to use as you observe your breath. But if you have the time, Richard says that practicing them all in order will make your breath become more "harmonious."

1. **Time.** Observe the natural lengths of your inhalations and exhalations. Initially, does your breath seem rapid or slow? And which seems longer, your inhalation or your exhalation, or are both around the same length? Simply paying attention to your breath in this way will tend to slow it down, which may quiet your mind and make you feel calmer.

2. **Texture.** Observe the texture of your breath as moves in and out of your torso. Is it smooth or rough? Is it even or ragged? Simply paying attention to the texture of your breath will tend to smooth it, which will help quiet your mind. That in turn may slow down your breath, smoothing it even more, which will quiet your brain even more, in a kind of feedback loop.

   You can monitor the texture of your breath by sensing internally as it moves through different parts of your body or by tuning in to the sound of your breath. If you are listening to your breath, as your breath becomes smoother, the sound will be consistent from beginning to end, with no sense of strain near the ends of your inhalations and exhalations.

3. **Space.** Observe the movements of your breath in your torso. You can either do this by sensing the movements internally or by placing your hands on your belly, ribs, and/or upper chest.

   To sense the movements internally, imagine that your torso, from groin to shoulders, is an empty container. As you inhale, observe where in that inner space your breath seems to penetrate and where it doesn't seem to penetrate. Simply paying attention to your breath in this way may cause your breath to move into areas where you don't usually sense it, usually your low pelvis, high chest, and back torso.

   If you want to use your hands to sense the movements of your breath, place fingertips on your lower belly below the navel, on your upper belly and lower ribs, or just below your collarbones. If you have time, Richard recommends combining all three as follows:

   Start by resting the fingertips of both hands lightly on your lower belly, just below your navel. First, just feel the touch of your fingertips on your belly. Then feel all your fingers moving with your breath, rising on your inhalation and descending on your exhalation. Finally, compare the movements of both hands: Is one moving faster or slower than the other? Breathe this way for a minute or more.

   Next, move your hands to your upper belly and lower ribs. Spread your palms and place your ring fingers and pinkies on your belly, and place your middle and index fingers on your lower ribs. Repeat the three-step sequence you used for your lower belly. Because the right side of your diaphragm has to push against your liver, it's not uncommon for your left hand to move faster than your right. Breathe this way for a minute or more.

Finally, move your hands so your fingertips touch just below your collarbones. Repeat the three-part sequence you used for your lower belly. If you like, you can help your breath move into this area by gently pushing your collarbones up toward your head on your inhalations and holding them high on your exhalations. Keep the hollow of your throat soft. Breathe this way for a minute or more.

After this practice, release your hands and observe your breath as it moves sequentially through your torso from the lower belly to the upper belly to the upper ribs on your inhalation and how this sequence is reversed on your exhalation.

4. **Rest.** Observe the natural pause at the end of your exhalations and your inhalations, when you are "resting" from the actions you take while inhaling and exhaling. Then, if you feel comfortable, allow yourself to linger in the pause after your next exhalation. If your throat, jaw, tongue, the back of your neck, or other areas feel tense, just notice that. Then watch your next inhalation building during your rest and "receive" your inhalation when it feels ready. Breathe this way for a minute or more and then return to your natural breath.[1]

If you have the time and want to do a calming breath practice after this, see Calming Breath Practice: Extending the Exhalation in chapter 7.

Coping Skill 2: Calming Yourself with Supported Inverted Poses

Although there isn't anything in this chapter I haven't tried, my personal go-to coping strategy when I'm going through any kind of difficulty, whether short-term or ongoing, is practicing supported inverted poses. I'll explain why below, but first you might be wondering, what is a supported inverted pose? Basically an inverted pose is any pose where your heart is higher than your head. And a supported inverted pose is one where you use props to make the inverted pose easier to stay in for an extended time. These include full inversions, where your heart is higher than your head and your legs are above your heart, such as Chair Shoulderstand (Salamba Sarvangasana), Supported Plow pose (Ardha Halasana), and Supported Legs Up the Wall pose (Viparita Karani).

Supported inverted poses also include partial inversions, where your heart is above your head but your legs are not above your heart, such as Supported Standing Forward Bend (Salamba Uttanasana), Supported Downward-Facing Dog pose (Salamba Adho Mukha Svanasana), and Supported Bridge pose (Salamba Setu Bandhasana). Because

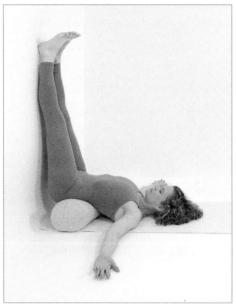

Full Inversion

you're standing on your feet in these poses, they tend to be a more active than the ones when your legs are not bearing your weight.

For a long time, all I knew was that I found these poses very calming. Then almost twenty years ago I took a workshop on the physiology of inverted poses from Iyengar Yoga teacher and sleep scientist Dr. Roger Cole that was a revelation. It's worth explaining what I learned because it will help you appreciate the effectiveness of these poses and also how to use them.

Roger explained that our bodies regulate our blood pressure based on our posture. That's because when we're standing or sitting up we need to be alert and ready for action, and when we're lying down it's time to either sleep or relax. So, when you sit or stand up after lying down, your body raises your blood pressure and stimulates your nervous system to prepare you for activity. And when you lie down, your body lowers your blood pressure, reduces your stress hormones, and calms you down because it's time to either sleep or relax.

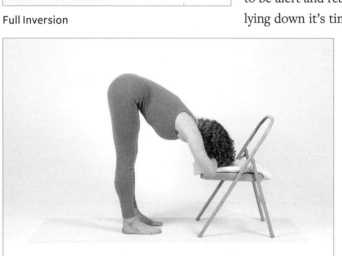

Partial Inversion

Our bodies know what "posture" we are in because of internal sensors, called baroreceptors, that are located in the artery above our hearts and in the main arteries at the sides of our neck. When blood flows away from your baroreceptors because your head is above your heart, they signal your brain and nervous system that it's time to raise your blood pressure and ready you to take physical or mental action. And when blood flows toward your baroreceptors because your head is at around the same level as your heart, they signal your brain and nervous system that it's time to lower your blood pressure and move you toward relaxation.

The wonderful thing is what happens when you do a yoga pose that is inverted (your head is below your heart). Because gravity causes even more blood to flow toward your heart and neck than would if you were lying flat, your baroreceptors send a stronger signal to your brain and nervous system. So your body more strongly lowers your blood pressure, reduces your stress hormones, and moves you toward relaxation than when you are just lying flat. Your position alone moves you into a deep state of relaxation!

The relaxing effects of being upside down don't take place immediately, however. I don't know of any scientific studies on this, but I've found it takes about 7 minutes for me to feel the full effects. So for practice during difficult times, I suggest 10 to 20 minutes so you relax completely and remain in that state for a good while. You can either do a single very comfortable pose, such as Supported Bridge pose or Supported Legs Up the Wall pose, for 10 to 20 minutes. Or you can do a series of poses for shorter times that add up to a total of 10 to 20 minutes, moving from one pose to another slowly and carefully to keep stimulation to a minimum.

Caution: Because going upside down causes blood to rush toward your head, inverted poses are not recommended for people with high blood pressure, glaucoma and other eye conditions, and other medical problems for which being upside down is contra-indicated. However, gentle inverted poses, such as a low Supported Bridge pose may be fine. If you have any concerns, I suggest you discuss this with your doctor before practicing them.

WHEN TO PRACTICE SUPPORTED INVERTED POSES

Because these poses are calming, you can do them any time of day or night, except right after a meal. They are especially helpful at the end of a busy day, such as after work and before bed. There is even a supported inverted pose you can do in bed if you can't sleep or are unwell: Supported Bridge pose with bent knees. Simply move the pillow that is under your head to be under your buttocks, and rest your head directly on the bed.

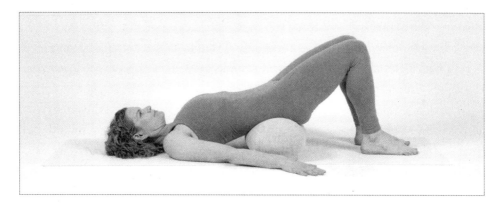

HOW TO PRACTICE SUPPORTED INVERTED POSES

You can practice any single supported inverted pose on its own, with the exceptions of Supported Shoulderstand and Supported Plow pose, which are usually followed by a pose that rests your neck, such as Legs Up the Wall pose—something I think makes good sense.

Here are the supported inverted poses I suggest for a single-pose practice. For all these poses, you can practice with eyes closed or eyes open with a soft gaze.

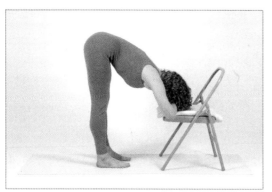

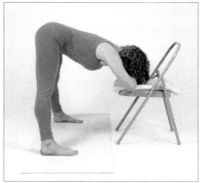

1. Supported Standing Forward Bend, *1 to 3 minutes*

2. Supported Wide-Legged Standing Forward Bend, *1 to 3 minutes*

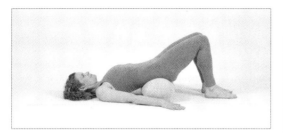

3. Supported Bridge pose, *3 to 10 minutes*

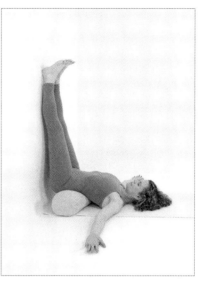

4. Supported Legs Up the Wall pose, *5 to 10 minutes*

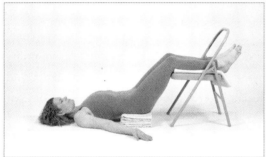

5. Easy Inverted pose, *5 to 10 minutes*

By the way, for those who don't already practice Supported Shoulderstand and Half Plow pose, I'm not going to include them in sequences in this book or describe how to practice them. That's because these poses can put stress on your neck, so I feel it's best to learn them under the guidance of an experienced teacher. I'm also not including Supported Downward-Facing Dog pose because getting the propping right for your particular body is a bit tricky, so that's also best to learn in person from an experienced teacher.

If you want to do multiple poses in a sequence, it's traditional to start with the partial, more active inverted poses before practicing the full, more relaxing poses. For example, you might begin with a Supported Standing Forward Bend or Supported Wide-Legged Standing Forward Bend (Salamba Prasarita Padottanasana) before practicing Legs Up the Wall pose. For a full sequence, see Evening Stress Management Practice on page 82.

Coping Skill 3: Resting Your Body and Mind with Savasana

The antidote to stress is relaxation. To relax is to rest deeply. This rest is different from sleep. Deep states of sleep include periods of dreaming that increase muscular tension, as well as other physiological signs of tension. Relaxation is a state in which there is no movement, no effort, and the brain is quiet.

—Judith Hanson Lasater, *Relax and Renew*

Sometimes dealing with change or living with a "new normal" makes you exhausted. And when you are contending with ongoing stress, you can easily become depleted. My husband and I both found that to be true for us during the early days of pandemic. Just our normal activities—working at our computers, doing housework, shopping for groceries—were more tiring than usual. We were sleeping well most nights, and he no longer had to commute, but still there were random times when we both got fatigue attacks.

And although not everyone likes to rest when they feel stressed out, many people do! And resting your body and mind while awake can be particularly beneficial because at the same time you are resting you are also de-stressing. Savasana is the perfect way to do this because this pose provides deep physical rest at the same time you rest your nervous system. The position you take for Savasana is a special one because this is the only yoga pose where your body is in anatomical neutral (or close to it). None of your muscles are stretching and none are contracting, so you can truly let go and rest completely. And if you practice a body scan, you can release physical tension from your body.

Savasana, by the way, is one of the few ancient yoga poses that we still practice in modern yoga. And from what I've read about the original practice, it was a reclined form of meditation. So, although Savasana is the name of the pose, it's also the practice that you do while you're in that pose, a practice that keeps you present physically and mentally while you are relaxing. To stay present throughout your time in the pose, you can use any mental focus, such as your breath, an image, a mantra, or a progressive physical relaxation, that you find easy to concentrate on. When you practice with a mental focus, you'll notice that even as your mind still wanders periodically, your thoughts will gradually slow down, and you'll feel calmer and quieter. This is a result of the relaxation response, which is triggered by your concentration practice. With time, you may even reach a deeper state of relaxation, in which you may feel as if you are floating, notice dreamy images flitting through your mind, or completely let go of your connection with external reality.

Because not everyone can get comfortable in the classic version of the pose, I'm going to start by offering you several variations you can try instead. I'll then provide information about the practice of Savasana.

SAVASANA VARIATIONS AND ALTERNATIVES

The purpose of Savasana is to enable you to rest completely, both physically and mentally. So that's why the position you take when you practice it should be comfortable, as symmetrical as possible, and relaxing. And, ideally, this position should be one where you do not need to use any effort to stay in the pose.

However, even though the classic version of this pose is very simple and takes no effort to maintain—you just lie on your back on the floor—many people find that this position isn't all that comfortable. For some, this might be due to a physical issue, such as back pain, tightness in the shoulders, or a stiff neck. Then there are those who aren't comfortable for emotional reasons: some people find lying flat on their backs makes them feel exposed or vulnerable. Whatever the reasons, if you're uncomfortable, you won't be able to experience the benefits of conscious relaxation. So if the pose isn't working for you, it's not working for you. There are also some people, such as those who are pregnant, who shouldn't be lying on their backs at all. Still other people tend to fall asleep in the classic position, and if you're sleeping in the pose, you're missing out on the benefits of conscious relaxation, which are quite different from sleep (although, of course, you need your sleep, too).

For all of you I just mentioned—and for anyone who would just like to be more comfortable in the pose—I'm offering seven different ways of practicing Savasana. Some are just slightly different than the classic version, and others are completely different. Be adventurous and give them all a try! You may even find that certain ones are better at different times. I myself practice version 2 in yoga classes and version 3 at home.

For all seven versions, feel free to cover yourself with a blanket, whether for warmth or a feeling of security. In general, if you're not comfortable in the pose, you won't be able to relax. So take the time to set yourself up with whatever props you like.

1. **Head support.** In this variation, you simply add a support under your head. This is beneficial for people who are tight in the shoulders or chest, who have stiff necks, or who find it uncomfortable to rest their heads on the ground. Most people benefit from a bit of support under their heads, so experiment to find what is right for you. Just make sure the support under your head is firm (not soft) and that your shoulders are touching the ground (not the support). Ideally in Savasana, your chin should be pointing slighting down toward your chest (not tipping back away from it).

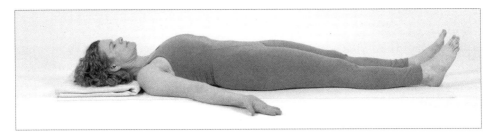

2. **Leg support.** In this variation, you use a prop under your knees. This is beneficial for people who have lower back problems or who simply want to rest their lower backs comfortably on the ground. Use a bolster (as shown below) or a rolled blanket under your knees.

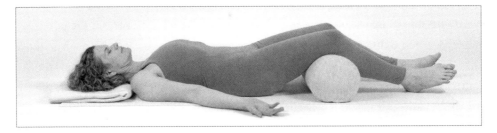

3. **Elevating your legs.** In this variation, you use a chair to support your calves, which allows you to relax your entire back on the floor. Because your legs are much higher than your torso, your position is inverted, which can enhance your ability to relax mentally as well as physically. If the seat of the chair is hard, place a blanket on it to make it cushier. When you settle into the pose, make sure that your legs are relaxed and drop comfortably onto the chair seat (if you are tall, you might have to stack blankets on the chair to make the surface high enough). If you can't get your legs through chair back, try turning the chair sideways instead.

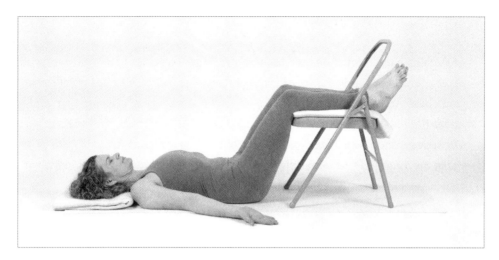

4. **Restorative Savasana.** In these two variations, you support your torso and head, so you are at an incline, with your head at the highest point and your feet at the lowest point. This position may be easier for you than lying flat on the floor or may even be deliciously comfy. Having your head above the level of your heart this way is slightly stimulating, so if you have trouble staying awake in Savasana this might be a good alternative for you. This supported position can also help you breathe more easily because the support helps open your chest. And it may make you feel less vulnerable than lying flat on the floor.

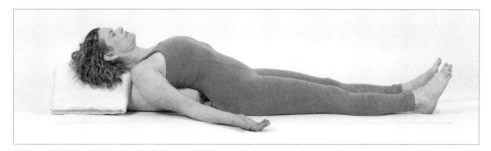

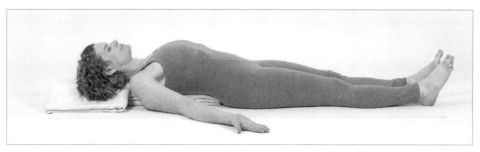

In the first restorative variation you use a bolster under your torso, and in the second you use a thin stack of two folded blankets instead. For both variations place a folded blanket or towel on top of the bolster or blanket stack to use for your head, making sure the support for your head is high enough so your chin can point toward your chest. After you set up your props, before you lie back, make sure that you sit on the floor in front of the bolster or blanket stack (not on the bolster or blankets). The support should be under your torso, but not under your buttocks!

5. Prone Savasana. In this variation, you take a prone position, on your belly, with your head supported by your forearms. This is sometimes called Crocodile pose (Makrasana). This alternative is helpful for people who feel anxious or vulnerable lying on their backs and need the comfort of having their front bodies protected. If this pose makes your lower back feel strained, try placing a blanket that is folded into a long, thin rectangle under your lower belly (below your navel) so your lower back doesn't arch as deeply.

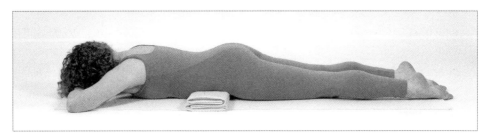

6. Side-lying Savasana. In this variation, you lie on your side with support under your head, between your arms, and between your legs. This is a good alternative for anyone who for any reason—medical or otherwise—cannot lie on their back or front. The supports between your legs and between your arms that are shown in the picture are important because they prevent your limbs from pressing together uncomfortably. You can use folded blankets or pillows as your supports, or any combination of the two.

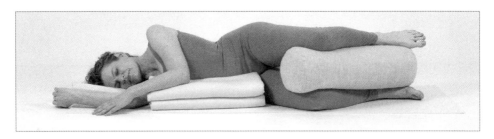

7. **Custom Savasana.** When you're practicing at home, be creative! If you don't have the props you want, try to see what else you have around the house that you can use. For example, could you use a couch cushion in place of a bolster, or could you rest your legs on an ottoman instead of a chair seat? And if there is something that hurts or feels uncomfortable when you're in the pose, see if you can figure out how to make yourself more comfortable. Like maybe when you lie on your back, your heels hurt a bit touching the hard floor. Could you use a folded blanket or towel to cushion them? Or put on special fuzzy socks? The deep relaxation you can experience from a good Savasana is worth putting a little extra effort into achieving. My friend Melitta recommends using an eye pillow—or, if you don't have one, a folded scarf over your eyes—and says that for her using this special prop "really makes for a deeper Savasana."

WHEN TO PRACTICE SAVASANA

You can practice Savasana anytime on its own—morning, noon, or night. And when you can't do an asana practice, such as when you are ill or injured, the ability to practice Savasana is always there for you.

If you have trouble sleeping, you can even practice Savasana after you go to bed, either before you fall asleep if you want to fall asleep more quickly or sleep more deeply or in the middle of the night if you wake up and can't fall back to sleep. However, if you want to practice a full session of Savasana for its special physical and mental benefits, it's best to do the practice when you're not sleepy because if you fall asleep in the middle of practice, you'll miss out on many of the benefits.

If you want to include Savasana in a practice with other poses, you can practice it at the very beginning, at the very end, or both.

HOW TO PRACTICE SAVASANA

The way you set up for and practice Savasana matters. Setting up so you're physically comfortable and symmetrical matters because being in physical discomfort, having objects in the room in contact with your body, and so on, distract you from your physical relaxation. And staying present throughout your practice matters because thoughts about the past or the future or about what's going on outside your practice room distract you from your mental relaxation (see below for tips about choosing a mental focus). However, when you start practicing, do your best not to judge yourself about how you are doing the pose because that interferes with your ability to relax. Simply let go of any judgmental thoughts when you notice them, and return to your Savasana practice.

Typically people practice Savasana with closed eyes, which helps you withdraw your sense of vision. However, if it makes you feel anxious or causes a downward spiral of depressive thoughts, you can practice with your eyes open. When you do practice with eyes open, try softening your gaze and looking slightly downward so you don't take in a lot of visual information about your surroundings.

If you have the time, I suggest you stay for at least 10 minutes in Savasana because it takes 7 or 8 minutes to trigger the relaxation response. Of course, you can stay even longer if you like. But if you don't have time to practice for 10 minutes, even a shorter Savasana can provide a welcome respite.

Here are some tips for maximizing your experience of Savasana:

1. **Set up your props carefully.** As you arrange your props, take the time to align them evenly and symmetrically. If you are using folded blankets, take care to fold them so there are no wrinkles, lumps, or uneven edges. And clear enough space in the room or on the bed so when you lie in the pose, you won't bump into furniture or stray objects.

2. **Stay warm.** If the room is cool, add extra layers to your yoga clothes, such as a sweater or shawl, and consider wearing socks. If that isn't warm enough, put a blanket or quilt next to you that you can use to cover yourself when you're in the pose.

3. **Align your body symmetrically.** After you enter the pose, take a few minutes to adjust your body, including your head, so it is as symmetrical as possible. If you are on your back, move your feet eight to ten inches away from each other and move your arms away from your body so your hands are six to eight inches from your body and your palms are facing up. Ideally, you don't want to feel one part of your body touching another part if that's possible in your chosen version of the pose.

4. **Consciously relax your body.** After you align your body, release it onto the support and encourage your muscles to let go of all activity. When you are in this neutral position, it's possible to relax your body completely. Then, commit to remaining still for the rest of your time in the pose. Remaining still helps quiet your mind as well as

your body by reducing external stimulation, which in turn tells your nervous system that you're safe.

5. **Withdraw your senses.** Sensory impressions stimulate your brain, so take a few moments to relax your sense organs. Rest your tongue on the floor of your mouth. Soften your eyes back toward your skull and, if your eyes are closed, gaze under your cheekbones. Finally, relax your ears, your nose, and your skin, consciously withdrawing your awareness from your senses of hearing, smell, and touch.

6. **Practice with a mental focus.** A mental focus helps you stay present in the pose, which allows you to experience conscious relaxation rather than being swept away by regrets over the past or worries about the future. It also helps you stay alert in the pose so you don't fall asleep. Options for focusing include:

   • Progressively relaxing individual parts of your body (sometimes called a body scan), usually starting with your toes and working your way up your body.
   • Practicing breath awareness (see Coping Skill 1: Centering Yourself with Breath Awareness on page 17).
   • Silently reciting a mantra (see How to Practice Concentration Meditation on page 208).
   • Picturing any peaceful image, such as a beautiful place in nature or a place where you felt relaxed and happy.

7. **Come out slowly.** Focus on moving slowly as you come out of the pose because quick movements are stimulating. You can start by opening your eyes just a crack, keeping your vision passive as you let the light fall into your eyes. Then ease back into movement by slowly wiggling your fingers and toes, and then maybe stretching your limbs a bit. Next, if you're on your back, you can slowly bend your knees and place the soles of your feet on the ground or on the prop you're using for your legs. Then, slowly turn over onto your right side and rest there for a couple of breaths.

   When you're ready to come to a seated position, instead of leading with your head, use your hands to slowly push yourself up to a seated position, with your head turned ww toward the floor until you are completely upright. Finally, when you are seated upright, slowly lift your head.

Coping Skill 4: Comforting Yourself with Restorative Yoga

You know how a small child will snuggle up with their favorite stuffed animal and special blankie when they need comforting? While restorative yoga was specially designed to provide you with deep rest and relaxation, many practitioners I know find it deeply comforting as well. Some even love their bolsters the way children love their blankies!

For those of you who are not familiar with restorative yoga, in restorative yoga poses you use props to support yourself in the shape of a classic yoga pose so you can be completely comfortable and completely relaxed, rather than feeling stretching sensations or muscular activity. For example, in Supported Child's pose, rather than folding forward all the way onto the floor, you use a bolster or stack of folded blankets to support your entire front body. The repertoire of restorative poses includes supported versions of classic reclined poses, forward bends, backbends, twists, and inverted poses. You can practice a single pose—Supported Reclined Cobbler's pose is a favorite choice—or include restorative poses at the end or the beginning of an active practice, or you can even practice an entire sequence of restorative poses.

If you're feeling anxious or vulnerable, prone poses (on your belly), such as Supported Child's pose, can be especially comforting. But if the pose alone doesn't provide the comfort you're seeking, you can try using a mental focus, such as your breath, while you're in the pose. This will signal your nervous system that you're now in safe circumstances, and it may help you relax more completely.

Because this section only provides a brief introduction to restorative yoga, if you fall in love with it and want to learn more, I suggest reading the books *Relax and Renew* and *Restore and Rebalance* by Judith Hanson Lasater.

WHEN TO PRACTICE RESTORATIVE YOGA

You can practice restorative yoga any time you wish, morning, noon, or night. You can even practice in bed when you're sick or injured. Some people even find it helpful to practice restorative poses, such as Child's pose, in the middle of the night when they're having trouble sleeping.

If you want to combine restorative poses with active yoga poses, typically the restorative poses would come at the end before the final Savasana. But if you're feeling fatigued you could begin with a restorative pose and then slowly ease into more active poses.

HOW TO PRACTICE RESTORATIVE YOGA

It's worthwhile to prepare for practicing restorative yoga. I suggest that before you set up your props, you start by creating a peaceful environment in the room where you are going to practice and change into clothes that will allow you to be comfortable and warm.

To create a peaceful environment, clear enough space in the room or on the bed so when you practice you won't bump into furniture or stray objects, and dim any bright lights. To dress for the practice, if the weather is cool, add extra layers over your yoga clothes, such as a sweater or shawl, because you'll cool down when you stay still, and consider wearing socks as well. You can also use a quilt or blanket to cover yourself after you're in the pose, whether for extra warmth or just for added comfort.

Now you're ready to set up your props. Because restorative yoga is all about being completely comfortable, the way you choose your props and the way you arrange them are important. So take the time to align your props symmetrically, and if you are using folded blankets, take care to fold them so there are no wrinkles, lumps, or uneven spots. Then, after you lie down in the pose, if you are not completely comfortable—if you feel muscles stretching or there is any physical discomfort—see if you can figure out how to change your props to make the pose work for you. And if you don't have the right props, you can use household objects such as books for blocks, towels for blankets, and bathrobe sashes for yoga straps instead.

When you are finally comfortable, you can choose whether or not to close your eyes. Closing your eyes helps you withdraw your sense of vision. However, if it makes you feel anxious or causes a downward spiral of depressive thoughts, you can practice with your eyes open. When you do practice with eyes open, try softening your gaze and looking slightly downward so that you don't take in a lot of visual information about your surroundings.

If the pose alone doesn't provide the comfort you're seeking, try using a mental focus. As in Savasana, using a mental focus helps you stay present in the pose, which allows you to experience conscious relaxation rather than being swept away by regrets over the past, worries about the future, or judgments about the present. It also helps you stay alert in the pose so you don't fall asleep. Options include:

- Progressively relaxing individual parts of your body (sometimes called a body scan), usually starting with your toes and working your way up your body.
- Practicing breath awareness (see Coping Skill 1: Centering Yourself with Breath Awareness on page 17).
- Silently reciting a mantra (see How to Practice Concentration Meditation on page 208).
- Picturing any peaceful image, such as a beautiful place in nature or place where you felt relaxed and happy.

The timing for restorative poses matters. You went through a lot of work to get into the pose, so staying for the minimum amount of time that I suggest below—unless you feel the pose isn't working for you—is worthwhile so you can receive all the benefits of the practice. On the other hand, staying too long in restorative poses, such as for hours at a time, can overstretch your muscles. So I suggest that you use a timer in this practice. A countdown timer on your phone will work well if you choose a pleasant-sounding alarm, but there are also special apps for meditation that have many different pleasant sounds you can choose from, such as chimes and gongs, that you might prefer instead.

When time is up, take a couple of deep soft breaths. As you come out of the pose, focus on coming out slowly, because quick movements are stimulating. The exact movements are different for each pose, but in each one see if you can use your hands to slowly push yourself up to a seated position instead of leading with your head or using your abdominal muscles. Finally, when you are seated upright, slowly lift your head.

Here are the restorative poses I suggest for a single-pose practice. For a sequence, see Afternoon Stress Management Practice in chapter 3.

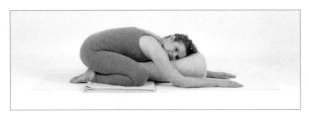

1. Supported Child's pose, from *90 seconds to 3 minutes per side*

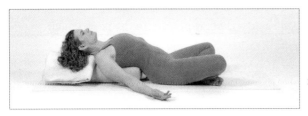

2. Reclined Crossed-Legs pose, from *5 to 20 minutes*

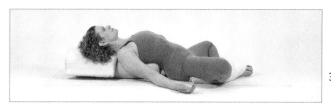

3. Reclined Cobbler's pose,
   from *5 to 20 minutes*

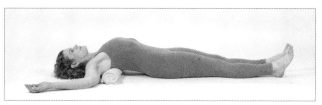

4. Supported Backbend,
   from *3 to 10 minutes*

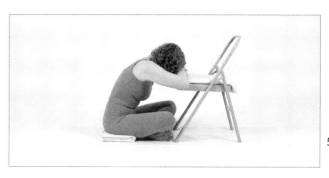

5. Easy Sitting Forward Bend,
   from *3 to 10 minutes*

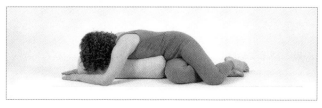

6. Supported Prone Twist, from
   90 seconds to 3 minutes per side

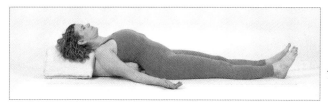

7. Supported Savasana,
   from *5 to 20 minutes*

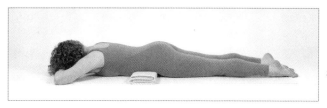

8. Prone Savasana,
   from *5 to 20 minutes*

Coping Skill 5: Taking a Break with a Mindful Asana Practice

Sometimes what's going on in the world or in your life is just too much, and you need some time out. But if your mind is racing or you have a lot of pent-up energy then relaxing, even with yoga, might not feel like the right thing to do. For times like these, an active yoga practice that engages your body as well as your mind can provide you with a brief respite.

In an active yoga practice, you always need to focus when you make the basic shapes of the poses and then come out of them, and as you stay in the poses, you need to focus to maintain your balance and refine your alignment. Using your concentration in this way helps anchor you in the present moment, which provides some respite from your regrets about the past and/or worries about the future. It can also help ground you when you're feeling distracted and scattered.

To enhance these benefits, you can use mindfulness techniques to transform your active yoga practice into a moving meditation. Practicing asana mindfully means finding a specific focus in your poses that will keep your mind engaged with your body. Then, as you practice, you move your mind away from your internal monologue and focus on what you're sensing in your body in the yoga pose. This helps steady your mind.

Yoga teachers often ask us to focus on the breath in our poses. This is an excellent technique because this traditional focus is simple and familiar. In a vinyasa-style practice, where you move in and out of poses with your breath, to coordinate your breathing with your movement you need to stay very focused. But you can easily do the same thing when practicing static poses by focusing on your breath both as you move in and out of the poses and while you hold them. However, focusing on the breath doesn't work for everyone because it makes some people tense or anxious to think about their breathing. And others may just want to try something fresh.

There are actually a surprising number of ways you can engage your mind and body with your senses in your yoga poses. My longtime teacher Donald Moyer used to give us very specific alignment instructions, often focusing on parts of the body we didn't usually think about, such as the piriformis muscle or the linea alba. The idea was that we would concentrate on moving that muscle or area of the body in a certain way—this alone was challenging if it was an area of the body you weren't used to moving—and then see how that "adjustment" affected the rest of the pose. Did it make the pose more comfortable or free up some energy? Or did it have the opposite effect? Donald even said: "Feeling an adjustment is concentration. Feeling the adjustment ripple through your body is meditation."

In Tantra Yoga, meditating on sensual experiences is both a way to be present in the here and now and a way to enhance your appreciation of the beauty of life in all of its fullness. In a mindful asana practice, we use our senses to experience our own bodies completely. They are so beautiful in all the different ways they allow us to experience our internal and external environments and to move through the world! Taking time to recognize all this in your asana practice can not only provide respite in times of difficulty or change but also encourage feelings of gratitude for just being alive to experience the fullness of life.

WHEN TO PRACTICE POSES MINDFULLY

Because I'm going to suggest practicing at least some challenging active poses for your yoga break—for most people active poses are the best ones for engaging your mind—I suggest taking a yoga "break" is best done in the daytime or early evening. This is because practicing active poses—especially standing poses and backbends—too close to bedtime can cause sleep problems. However, if the only time you can do this type of practice is when you're finally on your own at night, give it a try and see how it goes. Obviously, when there's a lot going on, any time you can manage a break is a good time to take it!

HOW TO PRACTICE POSES MINDFULLY

Although we typically think of our senses as being the classic five (sight, hearing, touch, smell, and taste), these are just the senses we use to interact with our external environment. We actually have three others, and these are the senses we use to tell what's happening inside our bodies. So, after I discuss how to choose poses for taking your yoga break, I'll provide information about two ways for you to engage your senses as you practice the poses in the sections called "Interacting with Your External Environment" and "Sensing Internally."

Choosing Poses and Sequences

For your yoga break, consider practicing at least some poses that naturally demand more focus: standing poses, balancing poses, vinyasas, and complex poses, such as twists, where you have to concentrate just to get into the pose. In addition, consider adding some level of challenge to your practice. While there is a time and place for a comfy, easy practice, this type of practice may not engage your mind as completely as one that is more physically demanding.

My colleague Dr. Ram Rao, who is a neuroscientist, Ayurvedic practitioner, yoga teacher, and author, says if you practice with the right level of challenge, you may even enter a "flow state," which is when your focus is undivided and you become completely involved in what you're doing, temporarily forgetting everything else. He explains this can happen when "one is engaged in an activity where the challenge matches the individual's skill, that is, when a person's skills are fully involved in overcoming a challenging task."

On the other hand, if your practice is too challenging (something I don't recommend doing anyway) that will lead more to frustration than being in the flow. So we're basically in Goldilocks territory, with you yourself needing to figure out what kind of practice is "just right" for you. And you might have to do some testing, as Goldilocks did. (If you haven't already done so, check the safety tips in the appendix. They will help you know when you should back off on the challenging poses or practices.)

In general, for all the poses you practice, practice mindfully as you go into the pose, stay in the pose, and come out of the pose. When your mind wanders, simply bring your attention back without judgment to your chosen focus.

Interacting with Your External Environment

Our five senses of sight, hearing, taste, smell, and touch provide us with the ability to interact with whatever environment we find ourselves in, whether indoors or outdoors. This is called exteroception. We don't typically use smell or taste in our asana practice—that I know of—but we can use our touch, sight, and hearing.

Touch. Your sense of touch provides you with awareness of how your body is interacting with whatever you are in physical contact with. This includes the surfaces you're touching—whether with your feet, hands, or any other body part—as well as how various parts of your body are interacting with each other. Here are some suggestions for how to use your sense of touch:

1. Observe how you're interacting with your props. For example, are you dropping onto a block or pressing lightly into it?
2. Focus on the surface that the foundation of your pose is touching (the foundation of the pose is whatever body part or parts are in contact with the floor or, for chair yoga, the chair seat and the floor). Can you feel the entire surface evenly, or is your weight unevenly distributed?
3. Focus on how two body parts are connecting, such as your raised foot and the inner thigh of your standing leg in Tree pose or the palms of your hands in Namaste.
4. Feel your breath. Sense your inhalations and exhalations as they pass through your nostrils. In poses where it is possible, you can use your hands on your belly, ribs, or upper chest to feel how your breath is affecting that part of your body.

Sight. Choose any visual focus in the room to concentrate on. This is a traditional practice of using a drishti (gaze) as a tool for concentration. You could also gaze at something in nature, such as a tree, a rock, or a flower, either when you're practicing outdoors or by looking through a window. But you may also find that maintaining a visual focus makes your balance steadier when you concentrate on a single point.

Hearing. Notice the sounds you make while you are moving in and out of poses or moving in a pose. Are you landing heavily with a thump? Or more gracefully and lightly? What happens if you try to be as quiet as possible?

Or, focus on the sound of your breath. You can even enhance the sound of your breath by slightly narrowing your throat. Then, use the sound of your breath as a gauge to tell whether or not your breath is smooth or jagged and uneven. If your breath isn't smooth, this can be a sign that you may be pushing yourself too hard. Can you make any adjustments in your pose to allow your breath to move more freely?

Internal Sensing

In general, internal sensing is a quieter way to practice than interacting with your external environment. That's because when you turn your awareness inward, it signals to your brain that you're safe, and that in turn triggers your relaxation response. We have three different internal senses: interoception, proprioception, and our vestibular system.

Interoception. This is our ability to feel what's happening inside our bodies. Interoception includes such things as sensing internally that your belly or chest is rising and falling with each breath, that your heart is racing or slowing, or that a muscle is activating, stretching, or relaxing. You can also experience an internal sense of energy flowing through your body in a pose (or getting stuck). Focusing on interoception is a very powerful practice. It helps keep you safe in a pose (pain can be a warning sign, and stretching in a joint area can cause injury), and for people with body-image issues it can help you learn to fully inhabit or "reclaim" the body you have. Here are some options:

1. Focus on how your inhalations and exhalations affect the rest of your body. As your lungs expand and contract, your body responds in various ways. You can focus on your upper chest, your ribs, your belly, your back, or even your pelvic floor area.

2. Focus on sensations of stretching in all your poses. Observe which muscles are stretching. And, for individual muscles, is the stretch in the belly of the muscle or at a joint? Is the sensation painful or just pleasantly stretchy?

3. Focus on the muscles you are contracting instead of stretching. Observe how you activate various muscles to move in and out of the pose. And when you're in a pose, observe whether there is some part of your body, such as your back leg or back arm, that you've been neglecting and that has gone limp or is collapsing? Balancing the activity of your muscles throughout your body will create a more even pose and can enable the energy to flow throughout your entire body. Also, check if there are any muscles that you are gripping too hard or contracting because you're feeling nervous or tense. Can you try intentionally relaxing that area? This can release blocked energy and create wonderful openings in your body.

Proprioception. This is an internal sense that allows you to feel where your body is in space. Proprioception is what allows you to walk in the dark (and what enables blind people to walk) and move the part of your body that is behind you without looking at it (like when you're getting in and out of a car), and it is an essential part of balancing. To observe this sense in action, close your eyes and bring your finger to your nose. You typically use proprioception to move in and out of yoga poses, such as when you position your back arm in Warrior 2 or step one foot back and turn the foot in for Warrior 1, and to make minor adjustments while in the pose. Here are some options for using it as your main focus:

1. Practice your poses with your eyes closed, so proprioception will be the only way you're aware of how your body is positioned. Doing balance poses this way is pretty interesting!

2. Focus your awareness on the parts of your body you can't see even with your eyes open, such as the back of your body.

3. Focus on your posture, which will help improve your posture in daily life as well as your proprioception. In every appropriate pose, while maintaining the natural curves of your spine, focus on elongating your spine and positioning your head directly over your spine—all without using your eyes. Or, use whatever cues you like for adjusting posture in your poses.

4. Use a single alignment cue you learned from a teacher as your mental focus for your entire practice, especially for parts of your body you cannot see. I like to focus on moving my shoulder blades the way my teacher Donald Moyer suggested, for example. Does it help you in some way? If yes, is it in all your poses or in only some? Can you figure out why?

Vestibular system. This is an internal sense you use for balancing in your everyday life as well as in yoga poses. It consists of three canals in your inner ears that provide your brain with information about the position of your body with respect to gravity, detecting whether the surface you are standing on is flat, such as a floor or a sidewalk, or uneven, such as a rocky path or a staircase. We typically practice yoga poses on a smooth, flat surface, but there are two ways you can focus on your vestibular system.

First, you can simply practice with your eyes closed, so as you move from pose to pose and as you practice any pose that involves an element of balance, you'll have to rely more on your vestibular system. You can also intentionally practice poses on an uneven or soft surface, such as on a folded blanket, a cushy carpet, or with your feet half on and half off a mat. Notice how this affects your ability to balance. A bonus is that practicing this way will actually improve your balance because balancing on uneven surfaces is essential in the real world. If you always wear shoes outside and walk on flat surfaces, your feet become less supple and responsive over time, so practicing yoga with bare feet on uneven surfaces can help your feet stay healthier and more responsive.

Brief Respite Practice

In this practice, focus on feeling your foundation—the parts of your body that are touching the floor—in all your poses. See if you can strengthen the foundation of each pose by pressing down toward the floor and from there extend your spine up (or away) from your foundation. If you practice Savasana at the end, as you sense which parts of your body are touching the floor and which are not, allow yourself to relax and release down toward the ground.

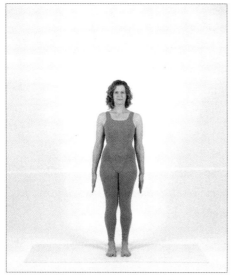

1. Mountain pose, *10 to 30 seconds*

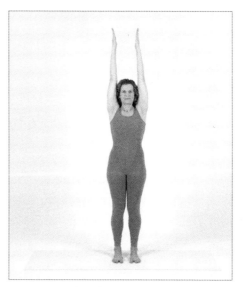

2. Arms Overhead pose, *30 to 60 seconds*

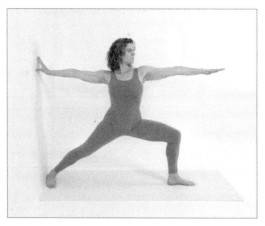

3. Warrior 2 pose, *30 to 60 seconds per side*

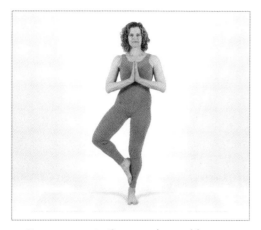

4. Tree pose, *30 to 60 seconds per side*

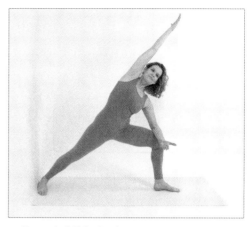

5. Extended Side-Angle pose,
    30 to 60 seconds per side

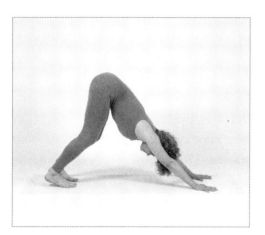

6. Downward-Facing Dog pose,
    30 to 60 seconds

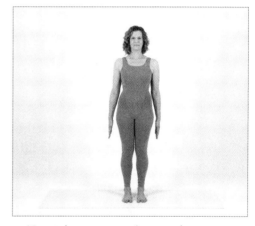

7. Mountain pose, *30 to 60 seconds*

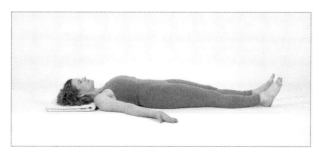

8. Optional Savasana

Coping Skill 6: Releasing Physical Tension by Stretching

My go-to practice to feel better, especially on a day when time is short, is to focus on hip and shoulder openers. Those are the big movement centers of the body, and I find that releasing muscle tension from those areas and keeping them mobile frees up a lot of energy. Feeling better in my body always elevates my mood as well.

—Sandy Blaine, positive psychology expert, longtime yoga teacher, and author

When you are feeling tense—typically from anger, fear, or anxiety—that tension can show up in your body as well as your mind. Your body can feel tight, stiff, or strained. I think this must be because we're on the alert and are holding ourselves ready to react with a fight-flight-or-freeze response. So your shoulders and/or legs may tense up. Sometimes this physical tension even shows up as minor aches and pains, such as neck pain, headaches, or back pain that are the result of tense shoulders.

One reason an active yoga practice makes you feel more relaxed is that a well-rounded asana practice does a great job of releasing physical tension from your body. Almost all yoga poses involve some amount of stretching, and stretching a muscle is what releases the tension from it. And often, when you release your physical tension through movement, it's such a relief that your mind, too, can relax.

So practicing yoga poses to release physical tension can be a good way to relax both your body and your mind! And you don't have to do a full yoga class or even a complete sequence to release your physical tension. One or two poses that target the area where you're feeling the tension may provide immediate relief. A bonus is that this type of practice also helps with stiffness and discomfort from long periods of standing or sitting.

Caution: Because back pain can have a number of different causes, if you're experiencing chronic back pain, I suggest you seek out a back-care yoga teacher, find a back-care yoga book, and/or check out some back-care videos.

WHEN TO RELEASE PHYSICAL TENSION

For most yoga coping skills, it's best to do a full session at one time rather than squeezing in bits and pieces throughout the day because it takes time to relax. But for releasing physical tension, even doing one pose as a little "yoga break" can help you feel more comfortable physically and mentally. And there are many stretching poses you can do in your street clothes, either standing up or sitting in a chair. So you can literally do a stretch or two almost anytime and anywhere, even a public place. I don't know about you, but I've done these types of poses at the airport and in waiting rooms, in the passenger seat of a car and in an airplane seat, in the back of an airplane during overnight flights, and in my office during the day when I worked at a software company. I'll provide some suggestions below for these kinds of poses.

However, if you have the time, you may wish to do a mini practice or even a full-length practice that includes poses to stretch different parts of your body for a more complete experience. In this case, any time of day is good, except perhaps just before bedtime because so many standing poses, twists, and backbends are stimulating and might be too energizing just before bed. If you do want to stretch just before bed, it's probably best to stick to a few gentle reclined stretches, such as Reclined Leg Stretch.

HOW TO RELEASE PHYSICAL TENSION

There are two basic ways to release physical tension. The first way is by holding a pose that actively stretches the muscles you want to release. For example, practicing a pose with your arms overhead, such as Arms Overhead pose (Urdhva Hastasana) or Half Downward-Facing Dog pose (Ardha Adho Mukha Svanasana), will stretch your shoulders.

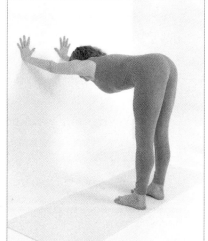

And a pose where you lift your leg toward your body or bend your torso toward your legs, such as Standing Forward Bend (Uttanasana) or Reclined Leg Stretch (Supta Padangusthasana), will stretch the backs of your legs.

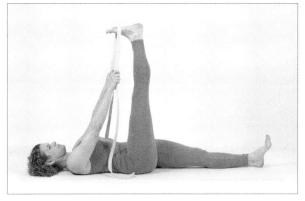

The second way is by slowly moving in and out of a pose that stretches the muscles you want to release. Moving in and out of a pose with your breath is called a mini vinyasa or a dynamic pose. For example, you would practice Arms Overhead pose by raising your arms overhead on an inhalation and lowering them on an exhalation. Repeating this movement several times can release tension from your shoulder muscles.

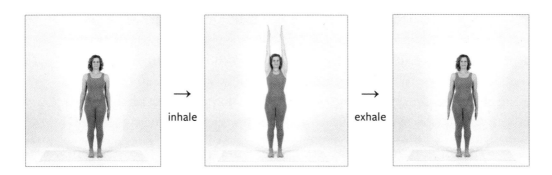

inhale   exhale

Likewise, you would practice Standing Forward Bend by moving into the pose on an exhalation and lifting back up to standing on an exhalation. Repeating this movement several times can release tension from the backs of your legs. If you practice this way, try to move slowly and gently, because moving (and breathing) too fast can overstimulate you and may cause your muscles to tense up rather than relax.

Depending on what you're comfortable with or enjoy the most, you can practice in either one of these styles or even combine the two. I typically practice static poses in the Iyengar style rather than as vinyasas, but I do often include the Cat-Cow (Marjaryasana Bitilasana) and Bridge pose (Setu Bandhasana) vinyasas in my sequences.

In both types of poses, be careful to keep your stretches gentle, backing off if you feel any pain (a mild stretchy sensation is fine). For static stretches, I suggest holding the stretch at least for 20 seconds because that's the minimum amount of time needed to trigger relaxation in a muscle. (If you want to improve your flexibility over time, try holding your poses for at least 90 seconds.) For dynamic stretches, I suggest six to eight repetitions.

When you practice a sequence of poses, I suggest you end your practice with a relaxing pose, such as Savasana, because relaxing physically can also help release physical tension, and this will counteract the stimulating effects of the active poses.

CHOOSING POSES FOR RELEASING PHYSICAL TENSION

In every single yoga pose except Mountain pose and Savasana, you are stretching some muscles while contracting some others. For example, if you step your feet wide apart for a standing pose, you're stretching your inner legs and contracting your outer legs. If you take your arms behind you, you're stretching the fronts of your shoulders while contracting the backs of them. And in twists, you're stretching one side of your body while contracting the other. So a balanced asana practice—with a mix of standing poses, forward bends, back-bends, twists, and inverted poses—will provide an all-over release for your body.

But if you want to target a certain area of your body, look for poses that stretch the areas that you want to release by studying the shapes of poses and/or feeling what is being stretched while you're practicing them. If you want a quieter stretch, choose seated or reclined poses. For more active stretching (or if you are in a place where you need to stand up), choose standing poses. If choosing by yourself feels intimidating, try my suggestions below, or ask your teacher for some recommendations. You can also look for articles or books that address how to stretch a certain area of your body, such as your hips, your back, your shoulders, and so on, and articles about office yoga or travel yoga have good tips for stretches you can do in public.

But because everyone is different—some people are naturally flexible, others are naturally less flexible, and others are naturally flexible in some parts of their bodies but not in others—you'll have to try the poses to see what works best for you. For example, some flexible people love seated forward bends for releasing their leg muscles, but if you're not particularly flexible in the backs of your legs, you may dislike these poses. So a better choice for you may be Reclined Leg Stretch, which might feel more comfortable for your back. Likewise, some flexible people may love Downward-Facing Dog pose for releasing their shoulder muscles, but those who are less flexible in the shoulders might struggle with this pose. In this case a better choice than Downward-Facing Dog pose would be a pose where you have your arms overhead but you don't bear weight on them, such as Arms Overhead pose.

Sometimes other body-type variations or even personal preferences can affect which poses you should choose. For example, some people may find twists helpful for back tension while others may prefer forward bends. So pay attention to your body as you try different poses. If you enjoy a pose and feel a gentle stretch in the area where you want to release tension, go for it. But if you feel uncomfortable in a pose—or just dislike it—try another pose instead.

SUGGESTED POSES FOR RELEASING PHYSICAL TENSION

Here are some suggested poses for releasing physical tension from specific areas of your body. You can practice one or two poses to target a specific area or you can practice some or all in the order shown below.

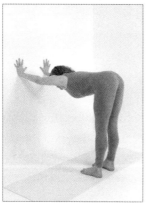

1. All-Around Stretch: Half Downward-Facing Dog pose, *30 to 90 seconds*

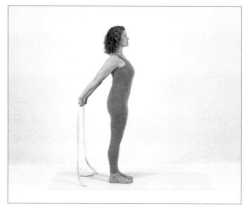

2. Shoulders: Standing Locust pose, *30 to 90 seconds*

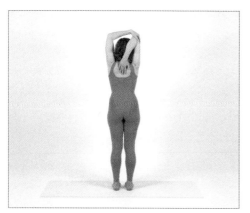

3. Shoulders: Standing Half-Cow Face pose, *30 to 90 seconds per side*

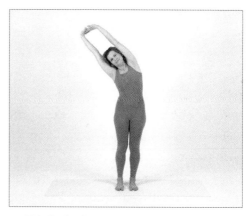

4. Side Body: Crescent Moon pose, *30 to 90 seconds per side*

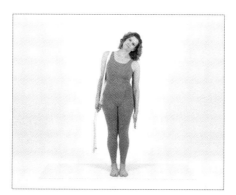

5. Neck: Sideways Mountain pose,
    30 to 90 seconds per side

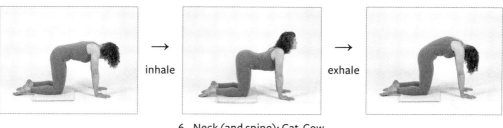

inhale   exhale

6. Neck (and spine): Cat-Cow
    pose, *6 to 12 repetitions*

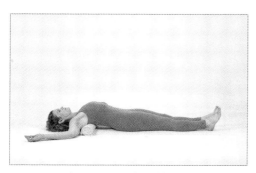

7. Front Body: Supported Backbend,
    3 to 5 minutes

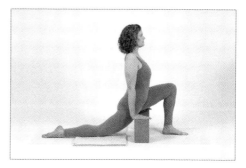

8. Legs: Dropped-Knee Lunge,
    30 to 90 seconds per side

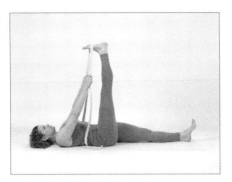

9. Legs: Reclined Leg Stretch 1,
    30 to 90 seconds per side

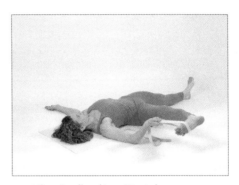

10. Hips: Reclined Leg Stretch 2,
    30 to 90 seconds per side

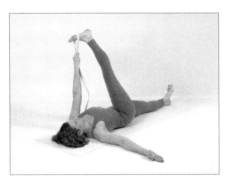

11. Hips: Reclined Leg Stretch 3,
    30 to 90 seconds per side

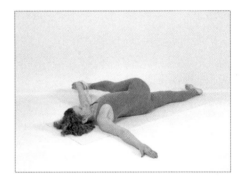

12. Hips: Reclined Twist,
    30 to 90 seconds per side

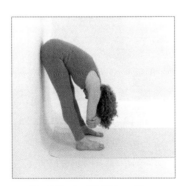

13. Back Body: Wall Standing
    Forward Bend, *1 to 3 minutes*

Coping Skill 7: Improving Your Sleep

Because insomnia is often the result of stress (your nervous system is keeping you awake and alert in case of emergency), all of the stress management techniques described in chapter 3 are a good start for improving your sleep overall. However, as I know from personal experience, when things are especially stressful there's a chance that even daily stress management practices won't help you much when you get into bed at night. That's because being alone with anxious thoughts when you're lying in bed in the dark can trigger your stress response again. The result is that you may have a hard time falling asleep initially, or, even if you do fall asleep quickly because you're exhausted, you may wake up in the middle of the night or in the very early morning and then be unable to fall back to sleep.

The good news is that there are yoga techniques you can practice while you're in bed that can help you to fall asleep or back to sleep. In addition, when you're going through a period of insomnia, you can plan your day as well as your night to support better sleep. The following sections provide suggestions for these two ways to improve your sleep.

WHEN YOU CAN'T SLEEP

This section provides a list of suggestions for practices you can do in bed, either when you're initially going to sleep at night or if you wake up in the middle of the night or very early morning and can't fall back to sleep. For those who are having trouble falling asleep initially, try one of the suggested practices as soon as you get into bed and settle into a comfortable position. For those who are waking in the middle of the night or early morning, try one when you wake up and realize you're not going to fall quickly back to sleep. If you are waking up in the middle of the night, consider practicing both before you go to sleep initially as well as in the middle of the night. Practicing before you sleep might help you sleep more soundly throughout the night because you'll fall asleep in a more relaxed state.

From this list, start by trying what appeals to you most or what you think will work the best in your current circumstances. If the first thing you try doesn't work or you just don't like it, try something else. Because it's often hard to think clearly in the middle of the night, you might even want to try out these techniques during the day so you are already familiar with them when you need them. When practicing any of these eight techniques, be sure to stay warm and keep the lights off to reduce external stimulation to a minimum.

1. **Breath awareness.** This is the easiest yogic breath practice and one of the most basic forms of meditation. It can help you fall asleep because it quiets your mind, and maintaining the practice for several minutes can trigger the relaxation response. See Coping Skill 1: Centering Yourself with Breath Awareness on page 17 for information on how to practice.

   If you use breath awareness as your meditation technique during the day, it's probably best to use another breath practice or another meditation practice (see Silently Reciting a Mantra just below) to fall asleep with. After all, during the day you want to stay awake when you meditate.

2. **Extending your exhalation.** This breath practice has two advantages over breath awareness. Exhalation lengthening takes more concentration than breath awareness, so your mind may wander less. And this practice has a special effect on your nervous system, automatically calming you down (see Calming Breath Practice: Extending the Exhalation in chapter 7).

   To practice, observe your natural breath for a few minutes as described earlier. Then, when you reach the end of your next exhalation, instead of immediately inhaling, lengthen your exhalation by one or two beats. Keep it relaxed, and if at any point you find the practice irritating, return to your natural breath.

3. **Other breath practices.** If there is another relaxing breath practice that you have experience with and that you enjoy, give that a try. See Breath Practices for Self-Regulation in chapter 7 for information about pranayama and how to decide which practices are relaxing, which are balancing, and which are actually stimulating and should be avoided at bedtime.

4. **Silently reciting a mantra.** Just as you would when you are meditating during the day, you can use a silent mantra or any word or phrase in bed to quiet your mind and keep yourself from spiraling into anxious thoughts. This is helpful for those of you who find focusing on your breath makes you anxious and for anyone who has a cold or another respiratory problem. See How to Practice Concentration Meditation in chapter 7 for information on mantras.

If you meditate regularly during the day with a mantra, it's probably best not to use the same mantra for falling asleep.

5. Guided relaxation. Following recorded audio instructions to guide you into physical relaxation—with or without earphones—focuses your mind on a soothing voice and on your physical sensations, which allows some to drift off to sleep. You could also try any guided meditation that is designed to help you sleep. If the person's voice or background music or imagery or anything else in a recording irritates you—yeah, that happens to me—look around for one that makes you comfortable instead. You may even find one recorded by someone whose voice automatically makes you feel calm.

6. Self-guided physical relaxation. When you are familiar with the basic instructions for deep physical relaxation, it's simple enough to skip the guided relaxation track and just gradually relax your body by following your own instructions. Many years ago, my first yoga teacher recommended this as an insomnia practice. And if there is any guided meditation that you've practiced often enough to memorize, you may be able to guide yourself through it in the middle of the night without playing the recording.

7. Slight inversion. A very relaxing pose you can practice in bed is a low version of Supported Bridge pose. This pose may be especially helpful because the gentle inversion naturally triggers the relaxation response due to your baroreflex (a mechanism in your body that helps regulate your blood pressure), so you don't need to focus on anything to make that happen. To practice, simply take the pillow out from under your head and lie on your back with your knees bent. Lift your pelvis up and place the pillow underneath your buttocks (but not under your lower back). If you wish, you can combine this with breath awareness or a mantra to quiet your mind as you relax. Try to stay in the position for at least ten minutes to give the baroreflex time to take effect and allow yourself to experience the full benefits of conscious relaxation.

8. Other restful poses. If you sleep alone or aren't worried about disturbing your partner, there are a few restorative yoga poses you can do in bed that have been recommended to me by practitioners who find them very helpful. Practice whichever appeals to you. If you want to combine them for a bed restorative session, I suggest the following order:

Supported Child's pose. Use two bed pillows to support your torso. Take your arms forward and hug the pillows or stack your hands on the top of the pillows to support your forehead, then slightly tug your forehead skin down toward your nose. Then bring your awareness to the back of your body and sense how your breath creates movement there, or practice any other form of breath awareness. Try to stay at least three minutes. If your head is turned to one side in the pose, switch to the other side when you're about halfway through.

Reclined Cobbler's pose or Reclined Crossed-Legs pose. Use your bed pillows to support your head and torso (but not your pelvis). If you are practicing Reclined Cobbler's pose and have two extra pillows, put one under each thigh. Bring your awareness to your belly and observe how your breath causes it to rise and fall, or practice any other form of breath awareness. Try to stay at least three minutes.

Supported Seated Forward Bends. Sit with your legs straight or in crossed-legs position (whichever is more comfortable and allows a deeper forward bend), and place a stack of pillows on top of your straight legs or in front of your crossed legs. Then lengthen your spine forward and rest your arms and forehead on the pillow and slightly tug your forehead skin down toward your nose. Bring your awareness to the back of your body and sense how your breath creates movement there, or practice any other form of breath awareness. Try to stay at least three minutes.

PLANNING YOUR DAY FOR BETTER SLEEP

If you have chronic insomnia and you don't already practice yoga at home, consider finding some time in the day or evening to practice yoga for stress management (see chapter 3). What you do during the day has an effect on the quality of your sleep at night, and keeping your overall stress levels as low as possible during waking hours can really make a difference in your sleep.

For those of you who do regularly practice yoga during the day or evening, I suggest you plan which yoga practices to do when. That's because while yoga in general is considered to be relaxing, some poses are more relaxing than others. And some poses and sequences, such as standing poses, backbends, and active flow sequences, are actually quite stimulating. If you jump into bed right after doing a stimulating yoga practice— or for that matter any stimulating form of exercise, such running, power walking, or

aerobics—it's sort of like drinking an espresso just before bedtime. Save those practices for earlier in the day.

For everyone, if you nap during the day, consider practicing relaxing yoga instead.
That may seem counterintuitive, but sleep, although necessary for your health, isn't
the same as relaxing while you are awake. Dreams can actually cause stress, as you have
probably noticed after waking up from a nightmare. And naps don't have the same
stress-reducing effects that conscious relaxation does. Unlike naps, conscious relaxation actually reduces your stress hormones, including your cortisol levels. Because
high levels of cortisol actually cause insomnia, lowering your cortisol levels with conscious relaxation or calming yoga poses could help prevent the busy mind and over-
stimulated nervous system that are keeping you awake at night.

Here are some suggestions for how to plan your twenty-four-hour day to improve
your sleep. Obviously, everyone's daily schedules are different, and not everyone has free
time during the day. So, if any of these suggestions don't work for you, just skip over them.

Daytime. Getting exercise is helpful for improving your sleep. So, if you have time
during the day to exercise, do the exercise that works best for you: walking, running,
swimming, cycling, doing aerobics, doing a strong yoga practice that includes force-
ful, stimulating poses, including standing poses, backbends, twists, and/or Sun Salutations and vinyasa flows, or taking an active yoga class from your favorite teacher. If
you're practicing yoga, however, try to end with a relaxing pose—whether that's Legs
Up the Wall pose or a good Savasana—so you quiet down after all the stimulation.

Afternoon sinking spell. Instead of napping during the day when you are sleepy, try a
conscious relaxation practice that won't put you to sleep, such as a seated meditation
or breath practice, or a restorative posture that you can do without falling asleep. Just
be sure to set a timer, perhaps one that chimes at intervals, in case you do fall asleep.
Another possibility is some gentle stretching, which is something you can do in the
same room with kids and pets—maybe they'll even join in (see Coping Skill 6: Releasing
Physical Tension by Stretching on page 48 for information about stretching).

Late afternoon/early evening. After work or the early evening is time for you to start
winding down and avoid stimulating poses and practices. You know how you stop
with the caffeinated drinks after three? It's like that. Additionally, many of us find our

stress levels peak at this time of day, so focusing on relaxing is especially beneficial. For people who practice yoga poses at this time, I suggest poses and practices that calm your nervous system, such as gentle stretches, forward bends, inverted poses, and/or restorative yoga. If this is a time when you take a yoga class, look for either a restorative yoga class or a gentle one.

Some people like meditating at this time of day because it helps reset them after a stressful day and make their evenings more peaceful, so doing that, or a calming breath practice, is also a good option. See chapter 3 for practices you can do to reduce your stress levels at this time of day.

Before bed. Sleep experts recommend going to bed at the same time each night. But before you go to bed, if it is at all possible, consider turning off the TV early or putting your book down and practicing a short yoga session to reduce your stress levels. Switching your nervous system to the rest-and-digest state before getting into bed may help you fall asleep more quickly and sleep more deeply. See chapter 3 for practices you can do to reduce your stress levels at this time of day.

It may even be that postponing bedtime by fifteen minutes in order to do a stress management pose or practice would be beneficial. You will not only be more relaxed when you get into bed, having a pre-bedtime routine might in itself be helpful, the same way that small children go to sleep more easily with a special routine that settles them down before bed. And if this is the only time in the day when you can do stress management practices, forgoing fifteen or twenty minutes of sleep to practice will also help keep your baseline stress levels lower overall.

In bed. For people suffering from insomnia, just getting into bed can trigger a new bout of stress. Practicing conscious relaxation in bed before falling asleep can help you fall asleep more quickly and/or help you sleep more deeply. So I suggest trying out coping skills 1 to 4.

In the middle of the night. All of us insomniacs are familiar with the terrible moment in the middle of the night when we realize we're wide awake and the possibility of returning to sleep feels hopeless. However, the worst thing you can do is lie there and worry about not falling back to sleep, because that just makes you more stressed out. Instead, return to the same practices you do before falling asleep. Although it takes some discipline to focus on these practices (for some reason, worrying seems like the easiest and most productive thing to do in the middle of the night), many people, including me, find that ten to twenty minutes of practice allows us to fall back to sleep. Sometimes it takes longer than that, I admit, but, at the very least, practicing yoga in bed gives you something more positive to do while you're awake than simply stressing out.

When Relaxing Isn't Relaxing

Did you ever do a yoga pose, breath practice, or meditation and start to realize that what it was supposed to be doing for you wasn't exactly taking place? Well, I certainly have; some types of pranayama that others find relaxing make me feel just awful. And I think it's essential for everyone to understand that traditional yoga relaxation techniques don't work for all of us. People are just very different from each other and have different things going on at any given time. For example, simple breath awareness is considered to be calming and a good way for a beginner to meditate. But some people, especially those with anxiety, find that focusing on their breath makes them feel panicky. And for people with depression, certain practices, such as meditation and yoga nidra, can even be dangerous because sitting or lying still with their eyes closed can send them into a downward spiral.

In addition, there are other purported benefits for particular yoga poses and practices that not everyone experiences. For example, supported forward bends may be quieting and soothing for many people, but for some they're aggravating or depressing. Likewise, backbends are traditionally considered uplifting, but for some they're agitating or just not effective.

So it's important for all of us to be honest with ourselves when we are not experiencing what we were expecting. And if you conclude that a practice is not working for you—it's not working for you! Once you acknowledge this, you can open up to some alternatives. The wonderful thing about yoga is that it is such a rich and varied tradition with so many different options and possibilities that there's a good chance that by exploring and experimenting you will find something that works for you.

Here are some suggestions for things to try when your relaxation techniques are not working for you. One good thing about these alternative techniques is that if you feel more relaxed, less anxious, or less depressed when you're practicing them, then they are working!

Keep eyes open. If closing your eyes in any pose or in meditation causes agitation or brooding, try keeping your eyes open but with a soft focus. Gaze downward instead of straight out at the world. Try opening your eyes fully, one half, or one quarter, and see what works best for you. These positions are actually traditional and are called full-moon eyes, half-moon eyes, and new-moon eyes.

Covering yourself. Sometimes lying on your back can make you feel exposed and vulnerable, especially when you're anxious. So, for Savasana or any restorative poses where you lie on your back, try covering yourself with a blanket. Sometimes that helps you feel more protected. If not, try practicing Prone Savasana (on your belly) instead. See Savasana Variations and Alternatives on page 29 for a photo.

Supported Child's pose. If classic restorative poses in which you lie on your back, such as Reclined Cobbler's pose, supported versions of Savasana, and Bridge pose with straight legs, make you feel exposed and vulnerable, practice Supported Child's pose instead. Many people actually find hugging their bolsters very comforting. You can turn your head to the side and keep your eyes open if that helps; just be sure to turn your head to the other side for an equal amount of time.

Supported inversions. Because these poses trigger the relaxation response owing to our basic physiology, if you're having trouble relaxing or concentrating, these are good alternatives to restorative yoga and meditation for rebalancing your nervous system (see Coping Skill 2: Calming Yourself with Supported Inverted Poses on page 23). You can keep your eyes open and even listen to relaxing music while practicing them, and you'll still quiet your nervous system. These are also great alternatives to seated forward bends, which cause some people to brood and others just find unpleasant. Of course, as with any pose, if you are uncomfortable in a supported inverted pose, come out immediately.

Choose appropriate breath practices. For some of us (like me!) breath practices have a very powerful effect on our nervous systems. So if doing a breath practice makes you feel uncomfortable in any way, either during or after the practice, I suggest you avoid it. Contrary to what you may have been told, not all breath practices are calming. Practices that encourage you to take a longer and/or deeper inhalation are stimulating and for some can actually be agitating. See Breath Practices for Self-Regulation on page 191 for how to choose appropriate breath practices. But if any breath practice—even a supposedly calming one—doesn't work for you, it's not working for you!

If no breath practices work for you, simple breath awareness as described earlier under Coping Skill 1: Centering Yourself with Breath Awareness on page 17 is an alternative. However, if focusing on the breath in any way makes you anxious, the solution is to do other things instead. Try meditating with a mantra or an image you hold in your mind rather than on a physical sensation in your body.

3

Stress Management for When You're Stressed

What happens to you when you are stressed out? Do you get headaches? Insomnia? Digestive problems? Are you short-tempered or anxious or depressed? Different people react to ongoing stress differently, but the symptoms are never fun, and in some cases they are actually dangerous, such as elevated blood pressure. Stress also affects the way you think as well as how you feel, and as a result—as you may have noticed—you may take actions or say things in the heat of the moment that you later regret. All of these are reasons why managing your stress levels is so important for adapting to and accepting change.

During 2020, I focused my yoga practice on stress management because I felt that staying balanced and steady through the fear and uncertainty was essential for me. So I committed to—as a minimum—meditating for twenty-five minutes and practicing Legs Up the Wall pose for twenty minutes per day. Some days I did additional yoga poses, some days I took a walk, and some days I did both. But I kept my commitment to myself and did my two stress management practices seven days a week. And when things got even worse because the state where I live went through an extreme fire season, I realized that, yes, these practices were working! Although I cared very much about people who were suffering as a result of these calamities, and I was concerned about the future of my state and of humanity as well as my own future, I was able to remain—most of the time—relatively calm.

This chapter is for those times in your life, times when you are experiencing stress day in and day out. This kind of stress can be a result of the state of the world or your community or just the state of your personal life. Either way, if you can change your circumstances, your yoga practice can help support you as you make those changes, and if circumstances are out of your control, your yoga practice can help you stay steadier as events unfold.

In chapter 1, I discussed some of the ways any change in our lives can cause "suffering." In this chapter, I'm going get a little more technical and describe how the stress you experience as a result of change affects your nervous system. I think it's important to understand a bit about how your nervous system works because yoga provides many different options for bringing your nervous system back into balance—or rather closer to balance because, yeah, sometimes you can only calm yourself down so much. Knowing what your options are and how they differ from each other will help you choose the best "yoga" for you when changes you're experiencing are causing you to stress out.

What Is Stress?

Basically, stress is a reaction to any significant change you experience. Because your usual routine might not be the most effective response to new circumstances, your nervous system makes you alert and prepares you to face a challenge. To prepare your body for action, your nervous system stimulates your heart to beat faster and stronger and slightly raises your blood pressure to improve your blood flow, and it opens your airways so you can breathe more easily. To prepare your mind for action, your nervous system stimulates your thought processes so that you focus, think more quickly, and assess your situation, and it heightens your emotions to ensure you respond with a sense of urgency. And the more significant the change is (in your mind, that is, since not everyone experiences the same types of changes in the same ways), the more your nervous system stimulates you and the more "stress" you experience.

By the way, even though we think of "stressors" as being negative changes, such as losing a job, ending an important relationship, or having your house or community destroyed by a natural disaster, all significant changes cause stress—even "happy" changes. For example, I remember after my first nerve-racking day at a job that I really wanted—working full-time on-site after a number of years of consulting from home—I just crawled home I was so exhausted, and I said to my husband jokingly, "Can I quit yet?" So whatever you find stressful is a stressor for you—it's good to admit that.

It's also important to recognize that stressors can include societal and environmental changes as well as personal ones. Of course, war, poverty, and discrimination—including racism, sexism, and homophobia—are stressors for those who experience them, as are the extreme weather, flooding, and long fire seasons caused by climate change. But even though we may not be personally affected by every change in our society, having empathy for the suffering of others can also cause us to feel stress.

Stress isn't necessarily a bad thing, however. It has an essential role to play in our lives since it prompts us to take action. But there's a big difference between acute stress, which you can recover from quite quickly, and chronic stress, which not only can continue for long periods of time but which can also take a long time to recover from. In the following section I'll discuss the differences between acute and chronic stress because even though you can use yoga to help reduce both types of stress, the best strategies for doing so also differ.

ACUTE AND CHRONIC STRESS

When you are facing danger, a threat of some kind, or a physical challenge, your nervous system triggers your stress response. This natural, healthy response prepares you to take immediate action. After all, even if we're not living in the wilderness, we still need to react quickly sometimes, such as to avoid an oncoming car or to stop a toddler from putting that pebble into their mouth. The stress response also helps you meet positive challenges, such as when you're playing a sport, performing for an audience, or brainstorming with another person.

This stress response that helps you meet an immediate challenge is called acute stress. It's a short-lived reaction, and after you have dealt with the challenge, you return to a state of balance. Your nervous system reduces the levels of stress hormones in your body, slows your heart rate, decreases blood pressure, reduces oxygen intake, and so on. Your body can then recuperate from the stressful experience. As you return to a state of balance, your racing mind will slow down, and you'll feel calmer. In chapter 2, I suggested many ways you can use yoga to recover more quickly from an episode of acute stress.

Chronic stress, on the other hand, is ongoing and never lets up. It is often caused by a change that completely disrupts your life, day in and day out. Some common examples are job pressures, marriage or family problems, and financial or health problems, as well as the societal stressors I mentioned earlier.

A good example of this type of chronic stress is what my husband, Brad, went through when he was finishing up his PhD at MIT. In addition to the pressure of completing his thesis on time and of then having to defend it, he was due to start a postdoctoral fellowship at Cambridge University immediately after that. So he and I also had to sell our apartment in Boston, put our things into storage, move to a city in England where we knew no one, and—oh yes, by the way—I was pregnant. During that period, he experienced heart palpitations and occasional panic attacks due to the ongoing stress. Even after we finally arrived, things continued to be stressful for him because we had to find a place to live on our own—which wasn't easy—and adjusting to English customs, ways of communicating, and ways of taking care of business was harder than you might think. He says now that it took him a full year to recover.

Although the stress you feel during these times isn't as intense as what you feel during an episode of acute stress, you never have a chance to return to a state of balance. Because your nervous system stays on the alert and ready for action, your body isn't able to rest and recover, and neither is your mind. That's why chronic stress can cause serious health problems, such as heart disease, hypertension, digestive disorders, headaches, and a weakened immune system. And it's also why chronic stress causes ongoing suffering, including emotional anguish as well as mental turmoil. The next two sections explain why.

STRESS AND YOUR EMOTIONS

Feelings play a very big role in shaping our perceptions and guiding us through life— bigger than most people realize.

—Robert Wright, *Why Buddhism Is True*

In *Why Buddhism Is True*, the psychologist Robert Wright explains that our feelings are primal responses that compel us as human animals to do what we need to survive and to protect ourselves and our families. Feelings of aversion, such as hate, fear, and anger, encourage us to avoid unpleasant or dangerous experiences. When we're particularly stressed out, our feelings of aversion, including fear, anger, anxiety, and depression, become more intense. The most intense stress response, your fight-flight-or-freeze response, is called that for a reason. You either feel anger so strong that it makes you want to fight or fear so great that you want to run or freeze.

In some high-stress situations, these feelings are actually helpful. For example, if you're out in nature in some areas of the world, you really might encounter a bear, a mountain lion, an alligator, or a poisonous snake. And in cities there are dangers, too, such as out-of-control drivers and people who are physically threatening you.

But in contemporary society, many very stressful situations are not actually life-threatening. When we experience acute stress while driving in traffic, performing, working on a deadline, taking a test, and so on, intense fight, flight, or freeze emotions are not useful. In fact, they can be counterproductive; we all know how stress can make us do things in the moment that we later regret.

And with chronic stress, you may experience anxiety, restlessness, lack of motivation or focus, irritability or anger, sadness or depression. Obviously, those feelings are not only unpleasant to experience but they can interfere with your ability to conduct yourself in a way that is in line with your values and goals. For example, if you're restless and irritated, it's hard to be patient with and loving to family members and friends or to work well with others. And for people who are susceptible, chronic stress can lead to full-blown emotional problems, including depression and anxiety, which can last long beyond the original incidents that caused the stress.

STRESS AND YOUR THOUGHTS

Perhaps you've noticed that when you're particularly stressed out, your mind races. That's because your stress response prompts you to rapidly assess your current situation, considering possible outcomes and solutions. But even more important is that stress affects the types of thoughts that you are having and the actions that you are considering.

Of course, our thoughts and feelings are very intertwined. In fact, according to Robert Wright, our primal and basic emotions are what trigger our thoughts. He says, "Every thought has a propellant, and that propellant is emotional."[1]

I discussed earlier how stress causes difficult emotions. Those emotions in turn can trigger thoughts that perpetuate your suffering. For example, someone with anxiety might constantly think about terrible things that might happen (this is called catastrophic thinking), or someone who is angry all the time might be obsessed with revenge fantasies. Those terrible thoughts may even cause you to say or do things you might regret afterward. I think we've all been there.

Because we typically have many different kinds of thoughts at a given time—some of which you might not even be aware of—when you are stressed, you may also be having thoughts that are more in line with your values and basic philosophy of life. But the strongest feelings you're experiencing and the thoughts those feelings have triggered can drown out more altruistic or compassionate thoughts that you might notice more when you're calmer. As Robert Wright says, "Feelings are, among other things, your brain's way of labeling the importance of your thoughts."[2]

I think that's why when we are in the fight-flight-or-freeze state, we tend to focus on fight-or-flight strategies (defend, avoid, retaliate, and escape), something I learned from the psychologist Dr. Dan Libby of the Veterans Yoga Project. In some situations, this high-stress thinking is appropriate. For example, a soldier in an actual battle needs to focus just on defending, avoiding, retaliating, and escaping, without other distracting thoughts. Likewise, this is true for you if your life is actually being threatened. But just as that form of high-stress thinking is not beneficial for a soldier in more peaceful situations, it doesn't work well for us civilians trying to get along with family, friends, neighbors, coworkers, and people in our communities. At times like these, we want to be able to consider altruistic and compassionate alternatives other than just thinking of "defend, avoid, retaliate, or escape."

In addition, for some, the thoughts triggered by intense emotions can cause them to get stuck in a cycle where a feeling generates thoughts that in turn generate more feelings. Dr. Scott Lauzé, who is a psychiatrist and mindfulness teacher, says that for some people with anxiety:

> Their mind thinks these thoughts, the thoughts then trigger a fear response, the sympathetic nervous system is activated, and that person is soon having a fight-flight-or-freeze response based on something that hasn't happened, and may not happen at all. It's a great example of faulty thinking-inducing suffering.[3]

So you can see why it's so important to manage your stress levels not only for your physical and emotional health but also to help you think more clearly during challenging times.

BRINGING YOUR NERVOUS SYSTEM INTO BALANCE

Thousands of years of self-study and experimentation led Indian yogis to discover many different ways to quiet their minds and bodies. Being in a state of equanimity was, for them, an essential step on the path to achieving liberation or enlightenment.

Traditionally, these practices were not called "stress management." However, modern scientists eventually provided us with explanations for how these techniques work: in different ways, they all trigger the relaxation response, a natural response that I described in chapter 2 that takes you into a state of relaxation, allowing you to rest, recover, and acquire new energy. (If you want more technical descriptions, I suggest you seek out information about the autonomic nervous system in general and how your vagus nerve activates your parasympathetic nervous system, the rest-and-digest side of your autonomic nervous system.)

Now, both in India and worldwide, these techniques are used to help us reduce stress and provide us with the benefits of conscious relaxation. With conscious relaxation (as opposed to sleep), you enter the rest-and-digest state. In this state, your body reduces your stress-hormone levels and returns to restoring itself, healing itself, and acquiring new sources of energy. Your emotional state shifts to feelings of peace and relaxation instead of the intense emotions associated with stress. And your mind gradually quiets, slowing down your racing thoughts and opening up to include different perspectives and ideas from the more limited options that you consider when you're stressed.

For acute stress, using these techniques can help you settle down after a stressful encounter and allow you to return more quickly to a state of balance. Perhaps you'll even be able to think more clearly about what just happened. And practicing these techniques on a regular basis can reduce your baseline stress levels so that when an incident sets off your stress response, you may not overreact.

For chronic stress, using these techniques on a regular basis can help lower your baseline stress levels. You'll not only feel better in the short term, but reducing chronic stress can also help prevent the serious illnesses and physical problems that it causes such as heart disease, hypertension (high blood pressure), digestive disorders, headaches, and a weakened immune system. And during times of change, reducing your baseline stress levels can be especially beneficial for your emotional and mental health, as lower stress levels can help prevent chronic anxiety or depression. Plus, when you're calmer, you may be able to be less impulsive and make choices that are more in line with your values and your goals in life.

In the next section, I'll provide an overview of the different techniques you can use to reduce your stress levels. I'll then make some suggestions for how to use these various techniques in your home practice.

Yoga Stress Management Practices

You can't directly tell your mind and body to "relax" the way you can tell your body to collapse onto a couch. However, by practicing yoga stress techniques, you send a message to your nervous system that you're now in safe circumstances. Your nervous system then takes the cue and triggers your relaxation response, moving you into the rest-and-digest state.

It takes a bit longer to "relax" this way than collapsing onto the couch, but in the end it's more effective than being a couch potato. Watching TV or getting lost in a social media feed are definitely distracting, but these activities don't provide the benefits of conscious relaxation, and sometimes—as you may have noticed—they even add to your stress.

Basically, yoga stress management practices fall into three categories: concentration practices, breath practices, and relaxing yoga poses. All together, there are quite a number of stress management practices so you have a good set of choices! The particular techniques you choose to practice should be based on your personal preference and what you find to be most effective. So here's an overview of the three types.

CONCENTRATION PRACTICES

Concentration practices are basically different forms of meditation. They trigger the relaxation response because you focus internally on something that isn't stressful to you. As you shift your awareness away from the outside world—and any problems it is causing you—as well as away from your worries about the future and/or regrets about the past, your nervous system triggers your relaxation response. There are three basic concentration practices.

Meditation. Yogic concentration meditation, in which you intentionally focus your awareness on your breath, on another physical sensation, or on a mantra, sound, or image, triggers the relaxation response. Even though your mind wanders and even if you feel like you're not doing a good job of meditating, when you repeatedly return your focus to your meditation object, your brain sends a message to your nervous system that you're now in safe circumstances. See chapter 7 for instructions on practicing this style of yogic meditation and for information about its other benefits.

Note that although mindfulness meditation, whether yogic or Buddhist, can help with stress in general, practicing it doesn't necessarily trigger the relaxation response because you may at times focus on painful emotions, thoughts, or physical sensations.

Savasana. This pose, which is called both Corpse pose and Relaxation pose in English, was traditionally a reclined form of meditation. In modern yoga, it is typically used to provide physical relaxation, frequently at the end of an asana practice. However, when you practice the pose with a mental focus, Savasana becomes a very powerful practice that can take you to deep levels of conscious relaxation. Because it is so powerful, I selected Savasana to be one of the coping skills in the previous chapter, one that you can practice on its own or as part of a sequence of yoga poses (see Coping Skill 3: Resting Your Body and Mind with Savasana on page 28).

However, some people find it hard to lie still when they are feeling stressed out. Doing an active yoga practice first might help with that. But if that doesn't help or you don't have time for it, try another stress management technique that is more active, such as supported inverted poses or seated breath practices.

Guided meditation. In this type of meditation, you follow instructions given by a teacher, either live or recorded, rather than practicing on your own. Some guided meditations, such as a body scan (described in chapter 2), focus on physical relaxation; some, such as the loving-kindness meditation, walk you through a formal meditation practice; and others, such as yoga nidra, combine the two. This way of practicing can be effective for people who have difficulty practicing on their own for whatever reason.

YOGIC BREATH PRACTICES (PRANAYAMA)

Yogic breath practices directly affect your nervous system by changing your heart rate. While not all breath practices are relaxing, practices that slow your breath or lengthen your exhalation will slow your heart rate, which in turn quiets your nervous system. So those two types of breath practices are good stress management practices. You can include these breath practices at the beginning or end of a session of yoga poses, before a meditation session, or at any time on their own. They're even good to practice in bed right when you turn in for the night or if you wake and can't fall back to sleep.

Because pranayama has so many other benefits, I will discuss it in depth in chapter 7.

YOGA POSES

Although many people—including many medical doctors!—think that all yoga poses are relaxing, there are quite a few poses, such as most standing poses and backbends, that are actually quite stimulating. However, yoga includes two types of poses that were specifically designed to be calming and to provide the benefits of conscious relaxation.

Restorative Yoga

As I mentioned in chapter 2, these modern yoga poses provide deep physical relaxation by supporting and relaxing your body. Many people find them comforting when they're worried or anxious, so that's why I included them as a coping skill. And if stress is making you feel fatigued, restorative poses can be especially helpful because they provide deep rest. If you use a mental focus while you're practicing restorative poses, such as focusing on your breath or the gradual relaxation of your body, you can intentionally trigger the relaxation response. So if you love restorative yoga, which many do, this can be a good option for stress management. See Afternoon Stress Management Practice on page 80 for a sequence.

However, some people find it hard to lie still in a restorative pose when they are stressed out. Doing an active practice first might help with that. But if that doesn't help or you don't have time for it, try another stress management technique that is more active, such as supported inverted poses or seated pranayama.

Supported Inverted Poses

Chapter 2 describes how modern supported inverted yoga poses—where you are either upside down or partially upside poses—trigger the relaxation response through the mechanisms that control your blood pressure. You don't need a mental focus (although you can use one) when you practice these poses. As long as you are warm, quiet, and comfortably supported in the pose, your nervous system will trigger your relaxation response after 10 to 20 minutes of practice (either in a single pose or in a combination of poses). Classic examples are Legs Up the Wall pose and Supported Bridge pose.

See Evening Stress Management Practice on page 82 for a sequence that includes several of these poses and Coping Skill 2: Calming Yourself with Supported Inverted Poses on page 23 for cautions about who should practice them.

How to Practice Yoga for Stress Management

If you want to use yoga to manage chronic stress as effectively as possible, it is worth taking the time to plan exactly what you're going to practice and when. The following three sections provide information to help you plan your day, your week, and the coming months.

CHOOSE WHAT'S RIGHT FOR YOU

Not every form of stress management works effectively for everyone. So choose the techniques that work best for you and your particular circumstances. If you already know that a certain technique doesn't work for you—for example, maybe you stress out as soon as you lie down in a restorative pose or sit down to meditate—just skip it. And if you try something for the first time and it makes you stress out more—or feel anxious or depressed—move on! My motto is: If it's not working for you now, it's not working for you now. You can always try again later, if you like.

Just make sure when you practice that you use seated or reclined positions that you can hold for extended periods of time so you can relax completely, and use appropriate propping to ensure you'll be entirely comfortable. If you're having a very hard time finding *anything* that works because, for example, just closing your eyes causes anxiety or depression, don't worry. This is more common than you might think, and I have some alternatives for you in chapter 2 under When Relaxing Isn't Relaxing.

Another issue to consider when choosing which techniques to use is what your aims are for your yoga practice. Are you just practicing to reduce stress? Or do you also want to follow steps along a particular yoga path?

The role of meditation in the traditional yoga paths is particularly important. Although you can use meditation for stress reduction, its role in traditional yoga is to quiet the mind completely—to cease all thoughts and feelings—as a way to achieve liberation or enlightenment. Pranayama is also an important component of traditional yoga, and it precedes meditation as one of eight steps on the path in Classical Yoga. It is considered an instrument to "steady the mind" and a gateway to *dharana* (concentration, the first phase of meditation). See chapter 7 for more information about both meditation and pranayama.

GIVE IT TIME

It takes time and regular practice to rebalance your nervous system and reduce your overall stress levels. So if this is your goal, I suggest you dedicate some time to it. If it seems like adding stress management to your already busy schedule is just too much, consider that if it makes the rest of your life better—which has been my experience— it's more than worth it.

In his book *The Relaxation Response*, Dr. Herbert Bensen recommends practicing for ten to twenty minutes to elicit the relaxation response. From my personal experience, it takes around seven or eight minutes of practice for me to feel the relaxation response kick in. After that, it makes sense to me to stay in that state for a good while to reap the benefits of conscious relaxation.

So, if you want to reduce your stress levels during a stressful period, I suggest practicing at least a short stress management session for about twenty minutes every single day, if possible. What you practice for your short stress management sessions could be any of the relaxation practices you prefer or that work in your current situation: seated or reclined meditation, calming breath practices, one or two restorative and/or supported inverted poses, or a guided relaxation program.

Because exercise is also important for reducing stress, you might want to supplement these relaxation sessions with an active asana practice or another type of exercise, such as walking, swimming, or cycling three or four days a week.

WHEN AND HOW TO PRACTICE

Guided relaxation, meditation, calming breath practices, restorative and supported inverted poses, and Savasana with a mental focus are practices that you can do on their own or include in a session of more active poses.

The most common way to include them in an active asana session is to practice them at the end of the session. However, you can also practice any of them at the beginning of the session to center yourself. And if you're fatigued, starting with a relaxing pose can be a good way to ease into the more active poses. But regardless of how you begin, it's always a good idea to "cool down" after your active poses with a quieting practice of some kind at the very end so you feel calm and relaxed after your session.

In addition, it's a good idea to practice your sequence of active poses in the daytime or early evening but not just before bed. That's because active poses, especially standing poses and backbends, can be very stimulating so it's best to avoid them just before going to sleep, even if you don't normally have insomnia.

For days when you just want to practice a short stress management session—whether you want to settle down after a stressful situation or just because that's all you have time for on a given day—you can choose any time of day to practice that works for you. If you're having trouble sleeping, however, practicing just before bed can be particularly helpful.

For many people, supported inverted poses are so effective for calming the nervous system and quieting the mind that even just one fifteen-minute session of Legs Up the Wall pose can turn the day around. And if these poses work well for you, then during your active practice days always include one or more near the end of your practice (before Savasana or meditation). Choose poses that you can hold for extended periods of time and use appropriate propping to ensure you'll be comfortable. Warming up for these poses with active or reclining poses that stretch your legs and open your shoulders may help you be less fidgety.

If stress is making you feel exhausted and depleted, consider putting together an entire sequence from restorative poses and/or supported inverted poses or perhaps combining them with gentle stretches.

If chronic stress is causing you to feel ongoing anger, anxiety, or depression, see chapter 4 for practices that target those conditions specifically.

Sequences for Stress Management

This section provides three different stress management practices that use different strategies. I'm calling them morning, afternoon, and evening practices because the most active practice is probably better to do earlier rather than later in the day if you are having trouble sleeping, and I thought a nice rest in the late afternoon might be good after a stressful day. However, you can practice any of these at any time of day. For example, if you're craving active poses in the afternoon, the morning practice would also work very well at that time of day.

Morning Stress Management Practice

This is a short active practice that prepares you to practice a long session of Legs Up the Wall pose. In the forward-bending poses, focus on bending from your hip joints while you keep your spine long. In Warrior 2 (Virabhadrasana 2), focus on keeping your torso centered over your pelvis and your head centered over your spine. In Triangle pose (Utthita Trikonasana) focus on keeping your spine long as you bend to the side from your hips. In Legs Up the Wall pose, find a neutral mental focus that helps you quiet your mind.

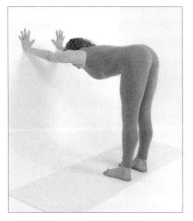

1. Half Downward-Facing Dog pose,
    30 to 60 seconds

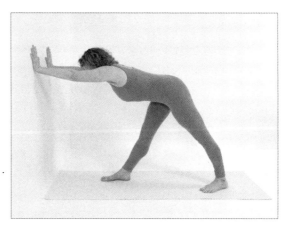

2. Half Pyramid pose, *30 to 60 seconds per side*

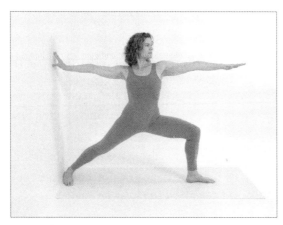

3. Warrior 2 pose, *30 to 90 seconds per side*

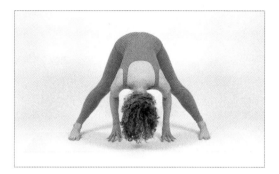

4. Wide-Legged Standing Forward Bend,
   30 to 90 seconds

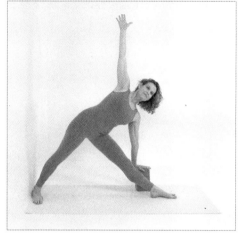

5. Triangle pose, *30 to 90 seconds per side*

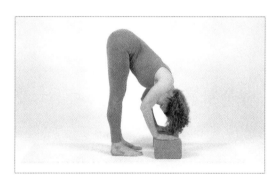

6. Standing Forward Bend, *30 to 90 seconds*

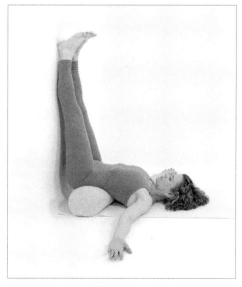

7. Legs Up the Wall pose, *10 to 20 minutes*

Afternoon Stress Management Practice

This is a resting sequence for when stress is making you feel fatigued. Skip any poses you don't like. In all the poses, you can focus on your physical relaxation, scanning your body for areas of tension and consciously releasing any you find with your exhalation.

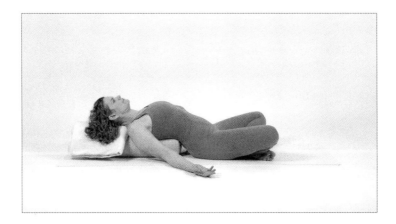

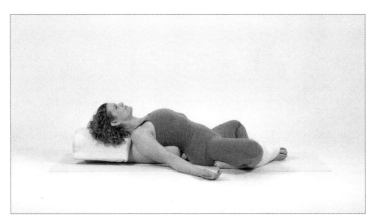

1. Reclined Crossed-Legs pose or
   Reclined Cobbler's pose, *5 to 10 minutes*

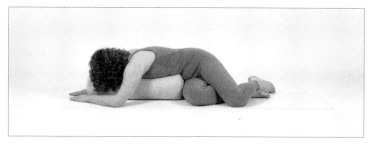

2. Supported Prone Twist, *90 seconds to 3 minutes per side*

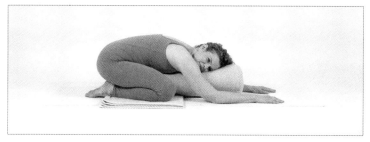

3. Supported Child's pose, *90 seconds to 3 minutes per side*

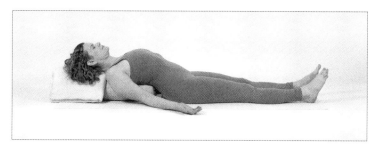

4. Supported Savasana, *5 to 20 minutes*

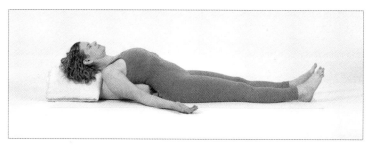

5. Optional breath practice: Equal Ratio Breath to balance your energy
   (see Balancing Breath Practice: Equal Ratio on page 198)

Evening Stress Management Practice

This sequence combines gentle stretches with gentle inverted poses. If you don't feel like stretching, just do poses 5–7. In poses 1–5, you can focus on relaxing areas of tension in your legs, shoulders, and hips. In poses 6 and 7, find a neutral mental focus that helps you quiet your mind.

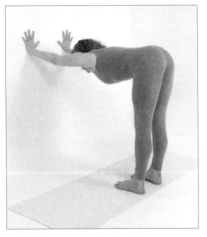

1. Half Downward-Facing Dog pose,
   30 to 60 seconds

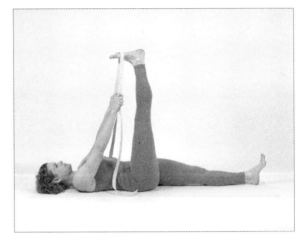

2. Reclined Leg Stretch 1,
   30 to 90 seconds per side

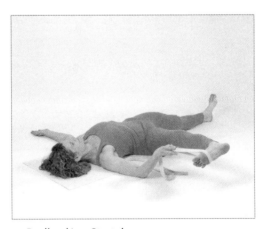

3. Reclined Leg Stretch 2,
   30 to 90 seconds per side

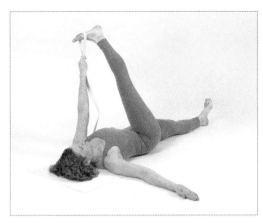

4. Reclined Leg Stretch 3,
    30 to 90 seconds per side

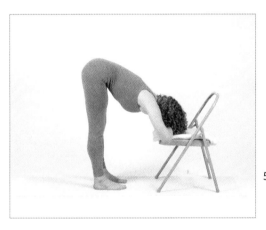

5. Supported Standing Forward Bend and/or
    Supported Wide-Legged Standing
    Forward Bend, *1 to 3 minutes*

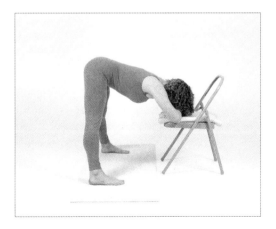

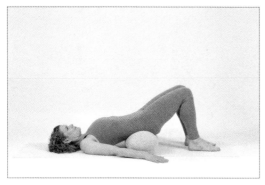

6. Supported Bridge pose, *3 to 10 minutes*

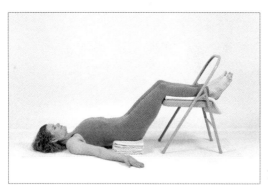

7. Easy Inverted pose, *5 to 20 minutes*

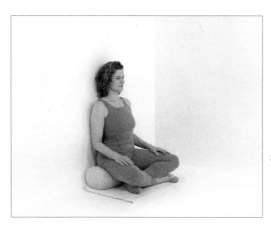

8. Optional breath practice: Extending
    the Exhalation for pre-bedtime calm
    (see Calming Breath Practice:
    Extending the Exhalation on page 197)

4

Moving Through Anger, Anxiety, and Depression

I started practicing yoga regularly when I was twenty-three, and in those days I was definitely lost and searching for answers. I used alcohol and drugs in an effort to handle my anxiety and the grief from dealing with so many friends who were sick and dying of AIDS. Yoga really saved my life. I can't imagine what would have happened if I hadn't gotten so involved with my practice back then.

—Jivana Heyman, yoga therapist, author,
and founder of Accessible Yoga

When you're going through difficult changes, it is normal to experience painful emotions, such as anger, fear, anxiety, and depression. As the yoga teacher and social activist Jivana Heyman describes above, as a gay man in San Francisco during the AIDS epidemic, he suffered from anxiety as well as from grief.

As painful as these emotions are, however, ignoring them isn't what will bring you peace. Instead, these emotions often function as important "signals" about your current situation that you should recognize and heed. As Jon Kabat-Zinn says in *Full Catastrophe Living*:

As with physical pain, our emotional pain is also trying to tell us something. It too is a messenger. Feelings have to be acknowledged, at least to ourselves. They have to be encountered and felt in all their force. There is no other way to the other side of them. If we ignore them, repress them, suppress them, or sublimate them, they fester and yield no resolution, no peace.[1]

In a Tantra tradition, all your thoughts and feelings are actually considered opportunities for you to learn about yourself rather than being "problems" that you need to fix. So accepting that painful emotions are natural and even beneficial at times may alone provide you with some relief from suffering. Because guilt and/or shame over having so-called "negative" emotions can compound the pain you're feeling, a good first step when you're feeling a surge of painful emotion can be to let go of any judgments about it (see Letting Go on page 234 for suggestions on ways to use yoga to release thoughts and emotions that aren't serving you).

The problem is that when you're in the throes of a painful emotion, it's not always possible to hear what it is telling you—not to mention that the painful emotion is just plain painful. So in this chapter I'm going to provide suggestions for how to use your yoga practice to reduce your emotional suffering, moving you more toward balance. It may then be easier for you to view your situation with more clarity and decide what actions you should take.

Because stressful situations are often what trigger painful emotions, I'm going to start with some background information about how painful emotions are often set off by our interactions with other people. I'll then introduce the general concept of making positive interventions for painful emotions with yoga. Finally, I'll discuss anger and resentment, fear and anxiety, and despair and depression individually, providing several different positive interventions for each of these specific emotions, along with suggestions about which signals each one might be sending you. I'll conclude with a general section on how to listen for the signals an emotion is sending and how to respond skillfully when you hear them.

As with the rest of the book, please consider everything in this chapter to be suggestions. If anything makes you feel worse, don't do it. And if a yoga practice or pose that I don't mention makes you feel better, go ahead and practice that!

Caution: For serious anxiety or depression, yoga should always be considered a supplementary treatment, not a stand-alone cure. You can use the techniques below to find some relief, to help you recover from a bout of anxiety or depression, or to prevent recurrence of anxiety or depression, but at the same time you should also follow the regime your health-care professional recommends, including taking medication if necessary. And please don't let anyone shame you—and don't shame yourself—if you need to combine yoga with medication. Instead, see if you can cultivate gratitude for all the things that are helping you, in both modern medicine and yoga.

If you're a yoga teacher and want to help someone who has serious anxiety or depression with some of these practices, always make sure the student is also under the care of a trained professional.

Stress Management and Painful Emotions

In chapter 3, I described how when we're particularly stressed out, our feelings of aversion become more intense, including fear, anger, anxiety, and depression. And I said that the most intense stress response, your fight-flight-or-freeze response, is called that because you either feel anger so strong it makes you want to fight or fear so great you want to run or freeze. Now I want to add that you might not realize how often we humans experience this powerful response.

Typically when we read about stress and the fight-flight-or-freeze response, there's an explanation of how for our hunter-gatherer ancestors this response prepared them to deal with large predators (tigers or mammoths or whatever) and other dangers in their outside environment. Then we read about how in modern times we typically don't face those types of dangers, but our fight-flight-or-freeze response is still triggered by less serious "dangers," such as a deadline at work or speaking in public. But it turns out that humans and chimpanzees have a more "active" fight-flight-or-freeze response than other primates, leading to a different explanation for why we still experience strong fight-flight-or-freeze responses on a regular basis.

Humans and chimpanzees are the only primates known to frequently engage in warfare. If this type of aggressive behavior was common during their evolution, then the fight-or-flight response likely played a critical role in adapting to the threat of deadly conflicts.[2]

Because humans and chimpanzees (unlike macaques and bonobos) tend to fight among themselves, some scientists theorized that our genes might reflect that we evolved to be on high alert from danger coming from our own species. And when they studied both human and chimpanzee genes compared to those of other primates, they did indeed find the evidence suggesting that "intergroup aggression" affected our evolution. This means that our strong fight-flight-or-freeze response could be genetically built in due to our tendency to fight each other and ultimately to conduct warfare.

After you get over the depressing thought that humans evolved to be better at fighting each other, it does explain some things. In the hunter-gatherer age, it wasn't just large predators that stressed us out on a regular basis, it was also other human beings! And guess who we are still surrounded by?

But even though human beings are our main stressors—not the growling dog or the rattlesnake—we also need other people in order to thrive. I think we learned both these lessons during the pandemic. We learned what being isolated from other people was like and how we missed them and needed them. And at the same time, we learned how other people, both loved ones and strangers, got on our nerves or worse when they did things we were averse to or that changed our lives in ways that made things harder for us. The stress all that caused was something many of us experienced as anger, anxiety, and/or depression.

All of this is why I feel it is important to focus on yoga stress management practices, such as those described in chapter 3, when you're suffering as the result of any painful emotion. Reducing overall stress levels can help moderate the effects of your stressful encounters with other people, helping you to think more clearly about possible actions to take, and it may also improve your relationships overall. In addition, because emotional disorders, including depression and anxiety, are either caused by or worsened by stress, practicing stress management for these conditions is very beneficial and may make you feel better, either immediately or with consistent practice over time.

However, emotional pain during times of change is a fact of life, and sometimes basic stress management only gets you so far. Fortunately, yoga also enables you to regulate moods and emotions individually, which can help you with anger, anxiety, and depression caused by stress or anything else. So when you find that basic stress management isn't doing the trick, combining it with a targeted approach to your emotional state can make all the difference.

POSITIVE INTERVENTIONS FOR PAINFUL EMOTIONS

In positive psychology, taking steps to regulate your emotions and increase your own well-being is called making "positive interventions." Sandy Blaine, a positive psychology expert as well as a longtime yoga teacher, says that positive interventions offer us some control over our own emotional states and may help us "ride emotional waves" more skillfully rather than simply reacting. And she says that yoga offers many different options for making positive interventions.

Yoga poses in particular can have a strong effect on your moods and emotions. I myself have been using my asana practice to regulate my emotions for around twenty years now, finding supported inverted poses very helpful for anxiety and backbends very helpful for mild depression. Although there are some general principles regarding the way that specific categories of poses will affect you—for example, that standing poses and backbends are generally stimulating and that inverted poses and forward bends are generally calming—the way a given pose will affect you as an individual may differ from the way it affects someone else. So in this chapter I'll provide a variety of suggestions for types of poses that could be helpful for anger, anxiety, and depression, and you can experiment to find out what works for you.

Yoga breath practices can also have strong effects on your moods and emotions. Calming breath practices can quiet your mind, slowing down the racing thoughts you can experience due to anger, fear, and anxiety. Balancing practices can be mildly calming or mildly stimulating, bringing you a feeling of stability. Stimulating practices may help energize you physically when you're feeling lethargic. See chapter 7 for complete information on how these practices work and when to choose which one.

Because we're all different, however, what works for one person may not work for another. So even though I have some specific suggestions below for the three different basic emotions, finding the best positive interventions for you will always be a matter of experimenting and observing.

HOW TO PRACTICE FOR EMOTIONAL WELL-BEING

During a period when you're experiencing anger, anxiety, or depression, it can be especially helpful to regularly practice yoga that specifically addresses what you're going through. This usually means practicing yoga at home instead of, or in addition to, attending a class or practicing with a video. So if you don't yet regularly practice yoga at home, consider starting, even if for only very short sessions of fifteen to twenty minutes, perhaps three days a week. And if you do practice at home already, consider practicing six days a week, even if only for very short sessions, during particularly difficult times. It may be challenging to begin a home practice when you're not already in the habit or to start practicing more often, but taking this important step to help yourself can be very empowering! You'll soon discover that there are healthy and safe things you can do to move yourself back toward emotional balance whenever you need to.

Anger and Resentment

I think we get confused in our practice and think that avoidance of uncomfortable feelings like anger leads to peace. But it doesn't work that way. Processing our feelings in healthy ways leads to peace. Anger can actually teach us a lot about ourselves. It may be a response to something that has challenged our worldview—our attachments.

—Jivana Heyman

When I discussed the fight-flight-or-freeze response earlier, I listed anger as one of the reactions you may experience as a result of stress. Changes that you are averse to can also make you angry, including changes that affect you personally, such as losing a job or someone ending an important relationship with you, and changes that affect people you care about or even society as a whole. As Dr. Lynn Somerstein, a yoga therapist and a psychoanalyst, said about the pandemic, "The future we had envisioned has disappeared, making us feel scared, cheated, bewildered, and angry as we fight against an invisible and implacable enemy."[3]

Although we tend to consider anger especially to be a "negative" emotion, it's actually a healthy signal that alerts us to a potential threat. Dr. Scott Lauzé says, "The way I think about it, anger is a normal response to certain situations, even a healthy one, and expressing that in a skillful way is normal and important."[4]

This form of aversion signals there is a potential threat that is physical, emotional, or both. And the threat could be to the well-being or survival of yourself, your family, others you love, or even to an organization, a community, or country that you care deeply about. When the threat is real, our emotion might be prompting us to try to find a possible solution to the problem. In *Real Change*, Sharon Salzberg says:

> When an interaction, person, or experience makes us angry, our bodies and minds are effectively having an emotional "immune" response. We are telling ourselves to self-protect, the same way blood rushes to the site of an insect bite. It is often anger that turns our heart-thudding distress into action, that pushes us to actively protect someone's right to be happy, to be healthy, to be whole.[5]

Yoga teacher and social activist Jivana Heyman says that love and compassion can be the basis for anger at witnessing someone causing harm. And that we can respond to this "righteous anger" by speaking out or defending the person or people who are being harmed. So anger at a real injustice or threat is not only a healthy response but can lead to beneficial acts and even to social activism.

But anger can also be triggered automatically as a result of patterns of behavior created by previous experiences that you've had. Yoga therapist Charissa Loftis says that she experienced anger on a regular basis when interacting with her family because of these types of patterns:

> I grew up in a home marked by PTSD, alcohol abuse, and depression. These issues heavily influenced our interactions with one another, and over the decades, those interactions shaped our habits and familial roles within the family.[6]

In addition, holding on to anger for too long—which causes you to cycle again and again through the same negative feelings and painful memories—can lead to a form of anger called resentment. Resentment not only doesn't resolve the conflicts you are reliving, but it can also cause you to experience what Sharon Salzberg calls "emotional bondage."

Dr. Lauzé describes resentment this way:

> We keep that little burning ember of anger alive and fan the flames from time to time. But, like a mentor told me, resentment is like lighting yourself on fire, hoping the other person dies of smoke inhalation. It ends up hurting us more than it hurts the other person, who frequently has forgotten all about the precipitating event and has moved on and has no idea you are harboring the resentment.[7]

Whatever situation you're facing, however, strong feelings of anger can make it hard to think clearly and use good judgment because you tend to focus on "fight" strategies prompted by your fight-flight-or-freeze response. So using yoga to cool down before making decisions is a good idea. You then may be able to navigate the situation facing you with more skill. Melitta Rorty says that to effectively deal with anger, she needs to observe it and figure out what underlies it. For her, this is almost always fear—which makes sense if you consider anger is often a reaction to danger just as fear is—and calming practices "give space to understand what lies beneath."

Yoga includes several positive interventions you can use to cool down when your anger is being triggered in the present moment. And for those who have ongoing problems with anger, yoga provides ways to reduce the intensity of this emotion so you can assess how to respond.

POSITIVE INTERVENTIONS FOR ANGER AND RESENTMENT

Dr. Lynn Somerstein told me that one winter day when she was walking down the street with her husband, her husband slipped and landed on top of her, breaking her ankle so badly that her foot was dislocated. He was unharmed. On her way to the hospital, she lay on the stretcher feeling like "the lowliest squashed worm." Later she realized that beneath her depression was strong anger at her husband. She said, "I was enraged and thought I might stay that way, but I didn't want to lose the relationship. I knew I had to forgive him." She said what helped her was "Pausing, feeling, accepting. Meditating. Chair yoga at first, then simple yoga on the mat."

The best positive interventions for anger will vary from person to person, depending on your particular situation, yoga experience, and personal preferences. Charissa Loftis says that she learned to use gentle yoga to "dissipate" the uncomfortable physical sensations her anger caused—the "hot boil" in her torso and face. Making herself more physically comfortable allowed her to feel the anger fully and to then let go of it more quickly than she had in the past. On the other hand, Iyengar Yoga teacher Jarvis Chen says that for some people active, full-body poses that engage all the large muscles of the body "can help the body to meet the energy of the mind and process the excess energy of anger."[8]

So you'll need to personalize your own approach by trying different strategies to see which work best for you. But in general, the poses and practices that people who have ongoing anger may find helpful include:

1. Standing poses. These poses can be grounding and help you burn off some of the excess energy that anger can cause.
2. Inverted poses. These are good for lowering your stress levels, which can tamp down the fight-flight-or-freeze response when you're too worked up for quieter practices. Inverted poses with head support, such as Supported Standing Forward Bend, Supported Wide-Legged Standing Forward Bend—and even Headstand (Sirsasana) and Shoulderstand (Salamba Sarvangasana) if you practice them—may be especially cooling for anger.
3. Demanding poses. Poses that fully engage your body, such as Downward-Facing Dog pose, Standing Forward Bend, and even Handstand (Adho Mukha Vrksasana) take you into the present moment and can interrupt the cycle of angry thoughts you are caught up in.
4. Gentle mini vinyasas. Moving in and out of gentle poses with your breath, as you do in Cat-Cow pose and a Bridge pose vinyasa, engages your mind and body while avoiding the stimulation some more vigorous practices can cause. Charissa told me that for her, moving with her breath was a "nice way to pull my thoughts out of 'the story' associated with the anger."
5. Calming breath practices. If and when you're able to sit still, calming breath practices can reduce your stress levels and quiet your mind. See Breath Practices for Self-Regulation on page 191 for more information.

There are also some poses and practices to consider avoiding when you're feeling angry. To start, Dr. Somerstein recommends that if you find a particular style of yoga stokes your anger, you should stay away from it. Other practices and poses you might want to avoid include:

1. **Stimulating breath practices.** Some yogic breath practices actually stimulate your nervous system rather than calming you, and these stimulating practices could increase your anger. See chapter 7 for more on these practices.
2. **Frustrating poses.** Poses that cause a lot of frustration or that you just dislike for whatever reason could increase your anger.
3. **Poses that cause brooding.** Poses where you turn inward, such as forward bends, or restorative poses where you feel like you are being left alone with your thoughts can cause some people to ruminate. If you have that experience and the pose increases your anger rather than reducing it, skip it for now.

RESPONDING IN THE MOMENT TO ANGER

If, in the midst of anger, you can't tell what the most skillful response would be, see if you can take a deep breath and stop for a "precious pause." This may give you a brief window in which to assess your current situation before reacting. If possible, use the meditation technique of "witnessing" what you're experiencing without any judgments. This is how Beth Gibbs described her experience with witnessing herself during a burst of anger:

> Physically, it felt like a volcano spewing boiling red lava in my belly. I noticed my breath. It was shallow and stuck in my chest. Energetically I felt heavy, tight, and constricted. Mentally, of course, I was seething.
>
> The act of witnessing was like being in the eye of a hurricane. It calmed me and I was able to watch my anger settle on its own.[9]

As Beth described, even just the process of bringing awareness to your anger can reduce its intensity. In her case, after her anger settled, she was able to act compassionately, rather than taking her anger out on someone who did not deserve it.

Dr. Lynn Somerstein, who describes herself as an "anger expert" because she grew up with people who were angry all the time and whose retaliatory rage caused her to hide her angry feelings, says that recognizing and "befriending" your anger is a good first step:

> Yoga brings you closer to your body, feelings, and mind. Thich Nhat Hanh said it best, "Breathing in, I know I am angry. Breathing out, I know that the anger is in me." The first step is to recognize and befriend your feelings, and then ask yourself why and how you are angry. Know that you are human, and the person you're angry with is human, too.[10]

But there are also a few other techniques you can use to reduce your anger so you can think more clearly about your situation and respond more skillfully to the situation you're facing. These techniques may even help you walk back from the edge if you feel like you might lose control.

1. **Focus on your exhalation.** After each inhalation, exhale consciously and deliberately, maybe even making a "positive" sound as you do so. These conscious exhalations may calm you down, and, as Iyengar Yoga teacher Jarvis Chen explains, because anger causes your diaphragm to tighten, conscious exhalations can help release that constriction.

2. **Rest your head.** It can be "cooling" to rest your head on a prop or on your hands. So if you're somewhere where you can sit at a desk or table, try moving your chair back a bit, bending forward from your hip joints, and resting your head on your hands for 3 to 10 minutes.

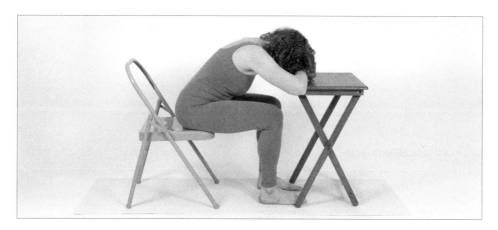

If you feel like you need to be more active, try Supported Wide-Legged Standing Forward Bend with your forearms and head on a table for 1 to 3 minutes.

Or, try practicing Supported Standing Forward Bend or Supported Wide-Legged Standing Forward Bend with a nearby chair for 1 to 3 minutes.

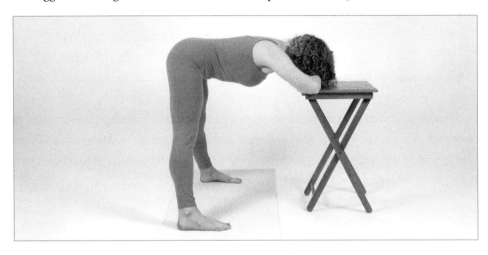

3. **Engage your body and mind in a full-body pose.** If you're somewhere where you can practice a yoga pose, try taking a break from the cycle of angry thoughts by practicing a pose that engages you completely, both physically and mentally, such as Downward-Facing Dog, Standing Forward Bend, or even Handstand (or a variation of it), for 30 seconds to 2 minutes.

Of course, if any of the coping mechanisms in chapter 2 are helpful in these circumstances, those are also good options for you. And if you have more time in the moment, you can do a longer practice, such as the Active Anger Practice on page 98 or Calming Anger Practice on page 100.

MOVING THROUGH ANGER OR RESENTMENT

Charissa Loftis, who described her dysfunctional family earlier, says that for many years she was trapped in a pattern of angry interactions with her parents. She says that after "lots and lots of yoga" as well as using Tara Brach's mindfulness technique called RAIN (a four-step process that includes "recognize, allow, investigate, and nurture"), she could see that the anger boiling up was "usually not a response to the current situation, but rather my family's long-held patterns of interacting with one another."

For those who have ongoing problems with anger and/or resentment, regularly practicing yoga's stress management poses can help you stay calmer overall and reduce your baseline stress levels. This in turn may mean you'll become angry less often or lose your temper less easily. I don't know about you, but I'm definitely more irritable when I'm stressed out. So that's why I think it's important in your regular practice either to focus entirely on stress management or to incorporate some of your favorite stress management practices into every sequence that you do.

In my calming sequence below, I'm suggesting practicing supported inverted poses for stress management because anger frequently makes you feel stimulated (ready to fight!), and these calming poses may be more accessible when you're feeling angry than quieter practices. But you can practice anything from chapter 3 that works for you for the stress management component of your practice. And if you can't practice inverted poses for any reason and think you'd like to try forward bends instead, try the Calming Fear and Anxiety Practice on page 113.

However, if you're really feeling worked up, you may want to start your practice with very active poses instead of stress management poses. This may help you dissipate some of your excess energy, which will allow you to settle down more easily when you practice your stress management poses afterward. That's why I'm providing both an "Active Anger Practice" and a "Calming Anger Practice" below. You can practice whichever one works best for you by itself, or practice them both, with the calming practice after the active practice.

If you find that very active poses fan the "heat and flames" of anger instead of dissipating your excess energy—as Charissa Loftis says was her experience—an alternative to a vigorous practice is to practice gentle poses where you move with your breath, such as Cat-Cow pose or moving into a seated twist on your exhalation and releasing on your inhalation. This brings the benefits of engaging your mind in the present moment while allowing you to release physical stress through movement. The Moving Through Grief Practice on page 162 is an example of this type of practice. You could practice this way before the Calming Anger Practice below or as a prelude to any stress management practices.

After practicing this way, if you're ready to "listen" to the signals your anger is sending you and consider skillful responses, see Listening and Responding to Painful Emotions on page 137.

Active Anger Practice

This sequence is designed to help you burn off some of your excess energy and bring your focus into your body and the present moment. In all the poses, focus on your exhalations.

If you want to lengthen the practice because you still have more energy, you could add in more standing poses before the Downward-Facing Dog pose or add in a mini Sun Salutation (Surya Namaskar) as shown in the Moving Through Grief Practice section in chapter 5 or a Sun Salutation of your choice before Warrior 1 (Virabhradasana 1). You could also repeat each of the active poses twice.

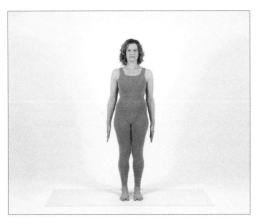

1. Mountain pose, *30 to 60 seconds*

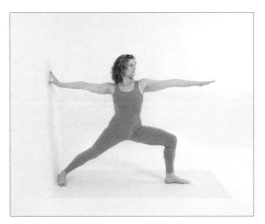

2. Warrior 2, *30 to 60 seconds per side*

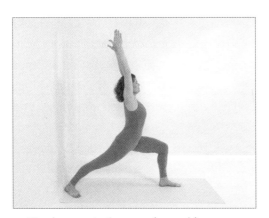

3. Warrior 1, *30 to 60 seconds per side*

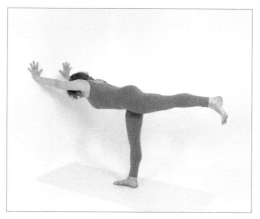

4. Warrior 3 (hands on wall),
30 to 60 seconds per side

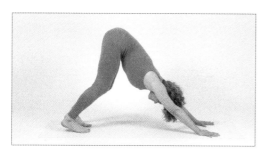

5. Downward-Facing Dog pose, *30 to 90 seconds*

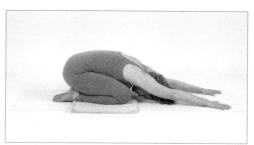

6. Child's pose, *30 to 90 seconds*

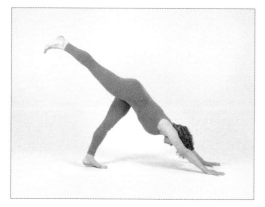

7. One-Legged Downward-Facing Dog pose
(or Handstand), *15 to 30 seconds per side*

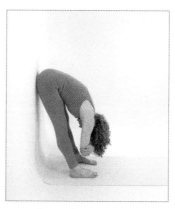

8. Wall Standing Forward Bend,
1 to 3 minutes

Calming Anger Practice

This sequence is designed to help you cool off and calm down. You can practice it on its own or do any active practice you like before it. In all the poses, focus on your exhalations.

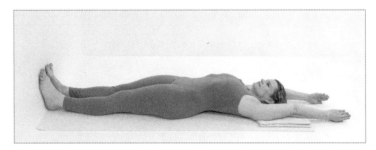

1. Reclined Arms Overhead pose, *30 to 90 seconds*

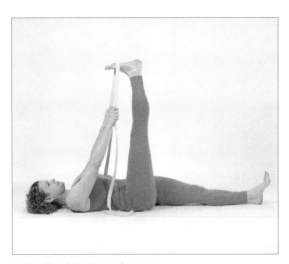

2. Reclined Leg Stretch 1,
    30 to 90 seconds per side

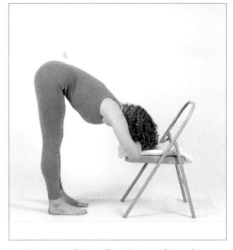

3. Supported Standing Forward Bend,
    1 to 3 minutes

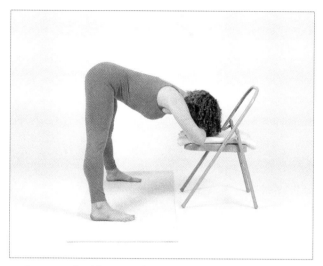

4. Supported Wide-Legged Standing
   Forward Bend, *1 to 3 minutes*

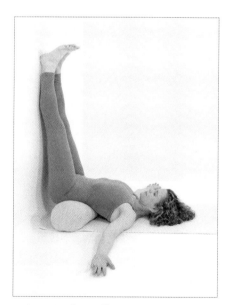

5. Legs Up the Wall pose, *5 to 20 minutes*

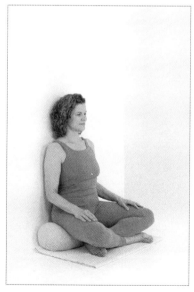

6. Optional calming breath (see
   Calming Breath Practice: Extending
   the Exhalation in chapter 7).

Fear and Anxiety

The emotion of fear arises with any threat to our well-being, whether physical, emotional, mental or spiritual. It can guide us to respond in a healthy way or, as we each
have experienced, entrap us in a trance of fear.

—Tara Brach, *Radical Acceptance: Embracing Your Life with the Heart of a Buddha*

Throughout her life, yoga teacher Nina Rook tended to experience anxiety, especially
during times of change. As a working mother before it was common in corporate life,
she already was spending whole nights running the same "what-if loops." Then, big
changes, including the end of her long marriage and the death of her older sister, made
what had once felt like "real and solid" plans for the future start to "melt away." Here's
how she describes that feeling:

> I saw family, friends, and colleagues visited by loss, sickness, and financial hard-
> ship in ways that seemed totally arbitrary. My long-term marriage dissolved,
> plunging me into the unknown and into bag lady fantasies. I dug myself out of
> the hole, built up my relationships with friends and family, and developed a
> vision of a future shared with my beloved older sister. And then, at 62, she died
> of an aneurysm. Again, I felt un-moored, with no clear path to a future.[11]

Anxiety and fear are very closely related. Anxiety combines your powerful urge to
plan with a constant fear that something terrible may happen in the future. This is
why anxiety is particularly associated with times of change—plans you already made
are no longer relevant, and the future is now uncertain. What if the worst is about to
happen? And when you have anxiety about the future, you may even be afraid of things
that might not even happen at all, becoming obsessed with making new plans based
on what-if scenarios, as Nina Rook did. And playing out these what-if scenarios in your
imagination can even increase your anxiety because your mind and body treat them as
if they're really happening. Dr. Scott Lauzé says that our amygdala, the part of our brain
responsible for triggering our fight-flight-or-freeze response, "responds to these imaginings even if they are not really happening or are unlikely to happen. To the amygdala,
they are really happening in that moment."[12]

But like anger, fear is a healthy signal. This form of aversion warns you that you or others you care about are in danger. As one of the emotions associated with the fight-flight-or-freeze response, fear can prompt you to take many different actions, including escaping, hiding, or freezing. Fear allows you to avoid real danger that is threatening you in the moment, such as by escaping from a burning building or ending an abusive relationship. And fear can also cause you to plan for the future, such as boarding up your windows in advance of a storm or putting aside money in an emergency fund.

However, both fear and anxiety can also stop you from doing things that are not actually dangerous, such as speaking in public or preparing your taxes. And, other times, your fear might be being triggered by memories of other frightening experiences that you've had. In *Radical Acceptance*, psychologist and Buddhist teacher Tara Brach describes it this way:

> Also part of our survival equipment, the emotion of fear is shaped by the accumulated experiences of our personal history. The affect of fear that arises in response to our immediate experiences combines with memories of associated past events and the affects they trigger. That's why some of us are terrified of things that hold no sense of danger for others.[13]

In all of these situations, the fear you feel may be preventing you from finding the most beneficial way of navigating the situation that you're facing. So for fear, like for anger, it's worth assessing whether the threat you feel is a real one and then, based on your assessment, finding ways to respond skillfully.

Responding skillfully to anxiety, however, may require a different strategy. That's because while for some anxiety is a mild, nagging sense of unease, for others it is serious, unrelenting, and can affect the way you think. As Dr. Lynn Somerstein says:

> An anxious person feels that they can barely stop themselves from falling apart. Many people experience jumpiness or hypervigilance, restlessness, sweatiness, the inability to concentrate, racing thoughts, unwanted thoughts, or fatigue.[14]

The inability to concentrate combined with racing thoughts obviously can make it hard to think clearly. In addition, anxiety can also cause physical problems, such as insomnia, digestive disorders, and headaches as well as emotional pain. So focusing first on calming down is a good idea because it will help with your physical symptoms as well as your ability to make good decisions.

Whatever situation you're facing, however, strong feelings of fear and anxiety can make it hard to think clearly and use good judgment because you tend to focus on "flight" strategies prompted by your fight-flight-or-freeze response. So using yoga to cool down before making decisions is a good idea. You then may be able to navigate the situation facing you with more skill.

Yoga includes techniques you can use to calm down when fear or anxiety is being triggered in the present moment. And for those who have ongoing problems with anxiety, yoga provides ways to reduce overall anxiety levels over time. I'll discuss these two scenarios separately below.

However, Dr. Lynn Somerstein says that for serious anxiety, if the feeling becomes your baseline after a few weeks, it's time for you to consult with a mental health worker, perhaps a therapist or psychiatrist. After that, you can use yoga in conjunction with the treatments recommended by your mental health professional.

POSITIVE INTERVENTIONS FOR FEAR AND ANXIETY

By chance I had two private students at the same time who were experiencing anxiety and panic attacks. Their life circumstances were very different as were their symptoms, so the programs I designed for them ended up being very different as well.

The first student's mother had recently died, after she had been at her mother's bedside in the hospital for weeks, and her panic attacks came when she was in bed in the middle of the night. After experimenting, we decided that the best technique for heading off a full-blown panic attack would be a breath practice where she consciously extended her exhalation. Although even just breath awareness can help with a panic attack or anxiety, having a specific exercise to do helped her focus more on her breath instead of just "watching" it. She later reported back to me, "The breathing has totally helped me, and it even helped me during the day when I was starting to freak out at a restaurant!"

For long-term relaxation, Legs Up the Wall pose was the supported inverted pose that suited her best. Since she was very active already with ballet lessons and wasn't a regular yoga practitioner, we decided that a mini practice of this one pose for ten to twenty minutes a day would be the best approach for her.

The second student had recently moved away from family and friends to go to graduate school. Her panic attacks came in the daytime, when she was fully awake and getting ready to face her day. She didn't want to try breath work because the thought of staying still to practice it made her feel even more anxious! Because she was hyper and restless, we decided she should try an active asana practice in the morning to head off the anxiety, followed by a short session of stress management with Supported Bridge pose, her supported inverted pose of choice, to reduce overall stress levels.

Because the best positive interventions for fear and anxiety will vary from person to person, you'll need to personalize your own approach by trying different strategies to see which works best for you. But in general, the poses and practices that people with anxiety and fear may find helpful include:

1. **Supported Prone poses.** Supported poses where you are facing the floor, such as Supported Child's pose and Prone Savasana, can make you feel safe and comforted. And if anxiety is making you feel fatigued, these and other restorative poses can provide deep rest.

2. **Forward bends.** Standing and/or seated forward bends can feel safe and quieting when you're anxious. There are some who find the classic versions of these poses challenging or unpleasant, but there are many ways to make forward bends accessible and even comfortable for most people, some of which are included in Calming Practice for Fear or Anxiety on page 113. So give these variations a try.

3. **Supported inverted poses.** These poses are particularly beneficial for anxiety because the physical orientation of the poses triggers the relaxation response, and concentration isn't as essential. They may also feel easier for you to practice than quieter forms of relaxation.

4. **Calming breath practices.** If and when you're able to sit still, calming breath practices can reduce your stress levels and quiet your mind. They may also be useful for heading off a spike in anxiety if you feel an attack coming on because they bring you into the present moment while also quieting your nervous system. See Breath Practices for Self-Regulation on page 191.

6. **Standing poses.** These poses can be grounding and help you burn off some of the excess energy that anxiety can cause.

7. **Moving with your breath.** Practicing gentle vinyasas, where you slowly move in and out of poses with your breath, can take you out of your anxiety and into the present moment and can uplift you emotionally when you're feeling overwhelmed.

8. **Stretching your hip joints.** In general, releasing physical tension as described under Coping Skill 6: Releasing Physical Tension by Stretching on page 48 can make you feel calmer as well as physically comfortable. Dr. Somerstein says that for anxiety and fear, stretching your hip joints in particular releases "stored bound energy," which might provide some relief. Hip openers include any standing poses or seated and reclined stretches where you take one leg out to the side, behind you, in front of you, or across the midline of your body.

There are some poses and practices you should consider avoiding when you're feeling anxious. In general, Dr. Somerstein recommends avoiding power or flow yoga when you're anxious because, she says, you can get swept up in a fast, difficult routine that might wind you up instead of down, and you might even get hurt. Other suggestions include:

1. **Stimulating breath practices.** Not all yogic breath practices are calming, and some forms actually stimulate your nervous system, which could increase your anxiety. See Breath Practices for Self-Regulation on page 191 for more information.

2. **Stimulating poses and practices.** Some challenging poses, deep backbends, and vinyasas that include jumping or moving quickly between poses can also raise stress levels and increase anxiety.

3. **Poses that feel unsafe.** Poses where you are supine (lying on your back), are tied up with a yoga strap, or have your eyes closed can make you feel vulnerable and increase anxiety. The same is true for poses that scare you, such as full inversions or deep backbends. So, as you practice any of the sequences in this book or any other sequences, whether in a class or on your own, be aware of how poses and practices affect you. If they're not working for you at this time, find an alternative.

4. **Meditation.** Although meditation is considered to be "calming," if you're feeling anxious, sitting alone with your thoughts could cause a downward spiral and make you feel worse. And Dr. Somerstein says that starting a practice on your own, especially when you're feeling anxious, is actually a bad idea. But if you already have a regular meditation practice and feel that the practice is helpful for your anxiety, then, of course, it's safe for you to continue practicing.

RESPONDING IN THE MOMENT TO FEAR OR ANXIETY

If you're not in immediate danger, such as from a fire or a car barreling toward you, see if you can take a deep breath and stop for a "precious pause." This may give you a brief window in which to assess your current situation before reacting. If possible, use the meditation technique of witnessing without judgment, which alone may help reduce the intensity of your feelings (see Meditation Basics on page 205). You may also want to take note of exactly what sent you near the edge (or over it) and what physical sensations you're experiencing because these are warning signs you may want to heed in the future.

If you have more than just a moment, there are several techniques you can use to reduce your fear and/or anxiety so you can think more clearly about your situation and respond more skillfully to what you're facing. These techniques may even help you walk back from the edge if you sense an anxiety or panic attack looming.

1. **Breath awareness.** This is the solution that I hear most frequently recommended for anxiety by a wide range of experts. As I described in chapter 2, breath awareness brings you into the present moment—out of your mind and into your body—and that may calm you down within a minute or two. As Nina Rook says, "The most powerful and immediate antidote for anxiety is simply breathing—when I focus on my breath, that focus disrupts and displaces the anxiety loops."[15]

   You can practice standing, seated, or lying down (either supine or prone). And you can combine this practice with the poses I suggest under numbers 3 and 4 below. For some, however, focusing on your breath can make you more anxious. For you it's better to do something else, such as reciting a mantra instead (see How to Practice Concentration Meditation on page 208) or practicing one of the yoga poses mentioned below.

2. **Seated Forward Bend at desk or table.** If there is a desk or table nearby, sit on a chair in front of it, bend forward from your hip joints—keeping your spine long—and rest your forehead on your folded arms on the desk. Try gently tugging your forehead skin down toward your eyebrows. Practice for 3 to 10 minutes. I confess I used to do this in my office when I worked at a software startup company back in the day, and it was very quieting. If you like, try sensing how your breath moves the back of your body.

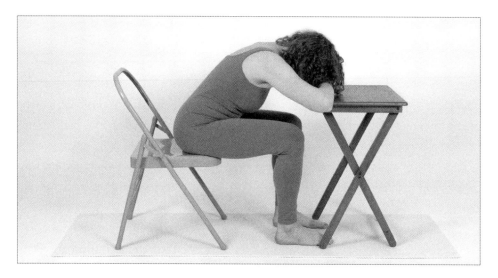

3. **Comforting prone poses.** If you're at home, you can try Supported Child's pose or Prone Savasana, either on your bed or on the floor. These poses can make you feel safe and comforted. Try gently tugging your forehead skin down toward your eyebrows. If you like, try sensing how your breath moves the back of your body. Practice Supported Child's pose for 90 seconds to 3 minutes per side and Prone Savasana for 5 to 10 minutes.

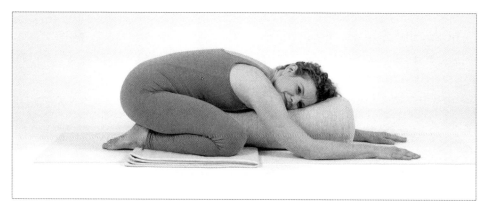

4. **Breath practices.** If you're comfortable practicing pranayama and already have experience practicing calming and/or balancing practices that work for you, these can be very effective for steadying you. See Breath Practices for Self-Regulation on page 191 for more information. However, if you don't have experience with pranayama, it's probably better to save this practice for when you're feeling more balanced.

Of course, if any of the coping skills mentioned in chapter 2 are helpful in these circumstances, those are also good options for you. And if you have more time in the moment, you can do a longer practice, such as the Calming Practice for Fear or Anxiety or Active Practice for Fear or Anxiety.

MOVING THROUGH FEAR OR ANXIETY

Looking back, I think it's something I've been dealing with on and off my whole life. The diagnosis made me realize how much yoga has been helping me all these years. I remember my practice giving me a sense of relief that I hadn't found any other way. It was such a powerful experience to find a way to address the suffering I was going through without drugs and alcohol. It definitely made me commit to yoga in a big way.

—Jivana Heyman

Jivana Heyman told me that he was diagnosed with an anxiety disorder a few years ago when he was having a particularly challenging time. His mother had just died and his teenaged daughter was getting into trouble. Along with his racing thoughts and a general feeling of being stressed and overwhelmed, he often felt like he couldn't breathe, clenched his teeth (and had associated headaches), and suffered from digestive issues.

The symptoms that Jivana described—both mental and physical—are very common for people with chronic anxiety as well as for people with chronic stress in general. So regularly practicing yoga for stress management when you have anxiety can improve your physical symptoms and enable you think more clearly. And because anxiety is caused by or worsened by chronic stress, practicing regularly can help you stay calmer overall and reduce your baseline stress levels in the long term. This in turn can help prevent anxiety and/or panic attacks from occurring in the future.

All of that is why I think it's important in your regular practice either to focus entirely on stress management or to incorporate some of your favorite stress management practices into every sequence that you do. At the beginning of the pandemic, I realized that my future was going to be filled with new challenges and dangers, and I felt it was a very high priority for me to stay as calm as possible. So I decided to change my yoga practice to focus primarily on stress management and to practice every single day. I'm happy to report that effort really paid off—I was able to stay relatively calm even through some challenging situations.

So if you, too, have had problems with anxiety in the past and find yourself confronting a situation that you are concerned will trigger your fear or anxiety, focusing on stress management practices ahead of time may help you maintain your equanimity as you face whatever comes next. You can practice anything that works for you from chapter 3 as the stress management component of your practice.

In the Calming Practice for Fear or Anxiety on page 113, I'm including forward bends combined with a supported inverted pose as a practice for anxiety because some people love the quieting qualities of forward bends. However, when you're in the throes of anxiety, you may have a hard time staying still for quieter poses and practices. Jivana found that was true for him, even though he was a longtime practitioner:

> It can be overwhelming to go from a place of stress or anxiety to complete stillness. There has to be a transition and a gentle way to go from that activity to the quietness. It reminds me of stopping a train that's going eighty miles an hour. You can't go from eighty to zero—that's crashing into a wall! Yoga offers techniques for putting on the brakes slowly, and that's what I started looking for.

So Jivana changed his practice during that period. Because he was too anxious to sit quietly in meditation or do subtle breath practices, he decided to practice more active and emotionally uplifting yoga poses, saying, "I think the more active asana practice helps to move energy in my body and leaves me feeling calmer."[16]

If you feel this way, too, a good way to make the transition to quieter activities is to start your practice with active poses, whether standing poses or moving with your breath, instead of stress management poses or practices. This may help you dissipate some of your excess energy, which will then allow you to settle down more easily when you practice your stress management poses afterward.

This is why I'm providing both an active practice for anxiety or fear and a calming practice for fear or anxiety below. You can practice whichever one works best for you by itself or practice them both, with the active practice coming before the calming practice.

After practicing this way, if you're ready to "listen" to the signals your fear and/or anxiety are sending you and to consider skillful responses to them, see Listening and Responding to Painful Emotions on page 137.

Active Practice for Fear or Anxiety

This sequence is designed to help you burn off some of your excess energy and to bring your focus into your body and the present moment, while also starting to calm you down. In all the poses, focus on feeling your feet (or feet and hands) pressing strongly into the earth.

If you want to lengthen the practice because you still have more energy, you could add in more standing poses after the Triangle pose or a mini Sun Salutation as shown in the Moving Through Grief Practice in chapter 5 before Warrior 2. You could also repeat each of the active poses twice.

After practicing this sequence, either move on to the Calming Practice for Fear or Anxiety that follows or simply add on any stress management practice of your choice—such as Legs Up the Wall pose or Savasana—to the end of this sequence for 10 to 15 minutes or longer.

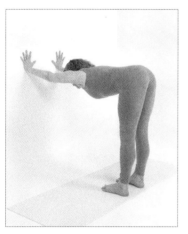

1. Half Downward-Facing Dog pose, *30 to 60 seconds*

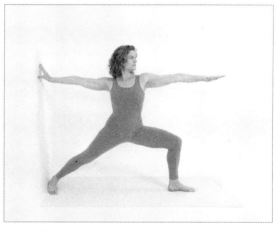

2. Warrior 2 pose, *30 to 60 seconds per side*

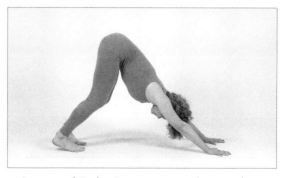

3. Downward-Facing Dog pose, *30 to 60 seconds*

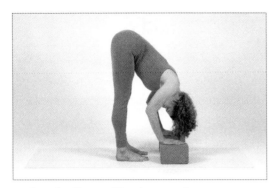

4. Standing Forward Bend, *1 to 2 minutes*

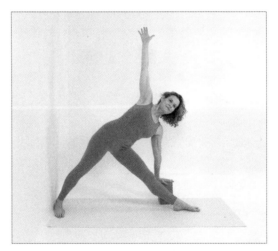

5. Triangle pose, *30 to 60 seconds per side*

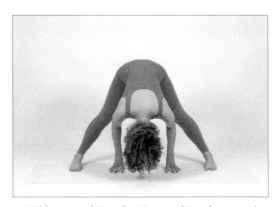

6. Wide-Legged Standing Forward Bend, *1 to 2 minutes*

Calming Practice for Fear or Anxiety

This practice focuses on forward-bending poses because they can be both comforting and quieting. Practicing all three seated forward bends will allow you to get the full benefits of the forward-bend experience because your time in the poses will add up. However, if there is one of these seated forward bends you much prefer, you could practice just that one but aim for holding it for a least 3 minutes. And if none of these poses work for you for whatever reason, you can try the Calming Anger Practice on page 100 instead.

In these poses, focus on bending from your hip joints and keeping your spine long as you also maintain the natural curve in your lower back. If the final pose makes you feel vulnerable, try covering yourself with a blanket.

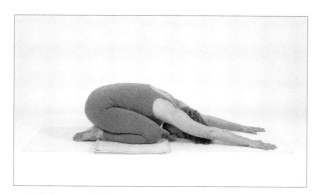

1. Child's pose (with extended arms), *1 to 2 minutes*

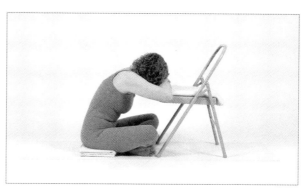

2. Supported Easy Sitting Forward Bend, *1 to 3 minutes*

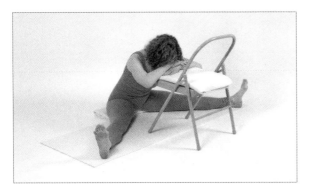

3. Supported Wide-Legged Seated Forward Bend,
    1 to 3 minutes

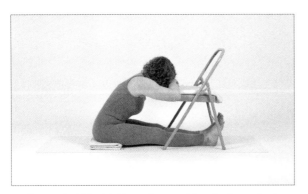

4. Supported Straight Legs Forward Bend, *1 to 3 minutes*

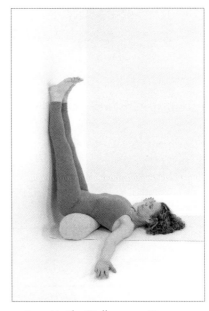

5. Legs Up the Wall pose or Easy
    Inverted pose, *5 to 20 minutes*

The Blues: Despair and Mild Depression

Although serious depression is a life-threatening mental illness, many of us experience mild depression and related emotions of discouragement and despair at one time or another. I remember that when my father decided to close his graphic design business so he could teach full-time, I watched my mother, who had helped him run his business, become depressed. She lost her appetite and took to staying alone in the bedroom for much of the time.

Dr. Somerstein says that symptoms of mild depression can include overeating or loss of appetite, difficulty sleeping or crying spells, feeling lethargic and numb, or experiencing irritability, outbursts of anger, or even violent reactions. They can also include problems with thinking and making decisions, lapses of memory, and feelings of guilt, worthlessness, and self-blame. I'll add that a particularly difficult symptom can be a feeling of hopelessness because you may feel stuck both in your life and in the feelings that you're experiencing.

We often feel mild depression, despair, or discouragement during times of change when we are comparing the present with the past and are feeling a loss. In my mother's case, she had lost not only her longtime job, which she loved, but her entire lifestyle as a woman working in the design field had come to an end. Eventually, though, she adapted to her new situation of being "retired" and found other activities to engage in. Then the depression lifted.

It's natural for us to remember the past and compare it to the present. In fact, our ability to remember is one of our greatest strengths as a species. And ruminating about the past can help us learn from our mistakes because we reflect on what happened, learn from what went wrong as well as from things that went well, and carry forward the lessons we learn. But even just remembering an upsetting incident from the past can trigger very strong emotions. Our brains are so effective at imagining the past that our nervous systems respond as if the events were happening in the present moment. So some of our ruminating about the past can churn up rather painful emotions.

In addition, depression can actually be a response to danger. Although there are differing opinions about what depression might be signaling, it is considered to be a form of "freeze" in the fight-flight-or-freeze response. Freezing can include immobilization (as in "playing dead") as well as hiding. Dr. Lauzé describes it this way:

In response to overwhelming stress, loss, or helplessness the sympathetic nervous system is triggered, and a person retreats as if into a cocoon, turning inward and away from the stressful environment and seeking safety by isolating (so as not be further hurt or disappointed), losing interest in external things (the outside world feels too scary), no longer feeling desire or joy (it feels too overwhelming to risk those things if they'll only be taken away), and sometimes sleeping for many hours a day (avoidance).[17]

The theory is that if your nervous system detects a threat that is so bad or that goes on for too long and fighting or fleeing aren't possible options, "freezing" is the only other possible response. I watched a friend go through this when the relationship they were in—one that they thought would be for life—became abusive. Because they still loved the other person, rather than ending the relationship or reaching out for help, they fell into a depression.

From this perspective, it's interesting that many people who are feeling depressed tend to have a similar forward-rounding posture, with a collapsed chest and shallow breathing. This makes sense because your "freeze" response could cause you to take a posture that protects your heart area and results in quiet breathing. In the yoga tradition, both changing the depressed posture by opening your chest and deepening your breath are techniques for improving your mood.

Depression may also be a signal that there is something wrong in your community or the world around you, such as climate change, income inequality, or racial injustice. In this case, taking action may be the best way to resolve your initial emotional response. As Dr. Timothy McCall says in *Yoga as Medicine*:

> Many people believe that if they feel sad, there is something wrong inside of them. But sometimes a depressed mood can be a healthy reaction to something that's not right in the external world, and dealing with it may be the best means of alleviating the depression.[18]

That is why for depression, as with anger and fear, it's worth assessing whether there is a real threat that is causing your emotional reaction. This could, in turn, lead to taking action, as my friend in the abusive relationship ultimately did. For community or

worldwide problems, even though you might not be able to solve the problem personally, you can take steps that will contribute to a solution in the long run.

But as with all these painful emotions, sometimes there is no appropriate action to
take. My mother couldn't get her job back—it wasn't right to ask my father to keep running a business that was stressing him out—and though she fantasized about ending
her marriage over the issue, that wasn't what she really wanted. Her depression was re-
solved when she accepted the new phase in her life. For those situations, making peace
with change might be the most skillful response.

Of course, it's hard to think clearly about whether or not to make change when
you're feeling depressed, and if you're feeling hopeless it can be hard to even contem-
plate change. Using yoga to uplift yourself emotionally, calm yourself, or both can be
helpful for thinking more clearly about what to do next while providing some relief from
some of your symptoms. And if you're feeling hopeless, taking even a small action, such
as practicing a yoga pose, can help you feel less "stuck" and allow you to feel a glimmer
of hope. Melitta Rorty, who has gone through bouts of depression after the end of a long-
term relationship as well as after being diagnosed with a chronic disease, says:

> I know that even just doing Legs Up the Wall pose can drastically change a bad
> "stuck" mood for me. So doing these self-care actions can be a springboard for
> change—you can feel the change however small, and that might give hope.[19]

Caution: Dr. Lynn Somerstein says that if your symptoms of mild depression last for
more than a couple of weeks and perhaps are worsening, you should find a psychother-
apist and/or certified yoga therapist to work with. And if your symptoms include cease-
less thoughts of death and suicide, if you have a family history of clinical depression,
or if you have experienced biological, sociological, or medical trauma that affects your
ability to feel, think, work, or be in a relationship, Lynn says that you might have clinical
depression. In this case, she recommends that you see a psychiatrist to determine what
course of action will help you.

TWO TYPES OF DEPRESSION

For all depression—even mild depression—there are two very different ways people
experience this emotion. In the yoga tradition, these two different forms are called
tamasic depression and *rajasic* depression.

The term *tamasic* comes from the Sanskrit word *tamas*. Tamas, one of the *gunas*—which are the three primordial qualities of matter that make up all of creation—is responsible for inertia. So tamasic depression is the type of depression where lethargy, fatigue, and hopelessness predominate. People with tamasic depression may have slumped shoulders, collapsed chests, and sunken eyes, and may seem as if they are barely breathing. Dr. Somerstein describes it this way:

> The first kind is a foggy sad state that we usually think of when we talk about depression—maybe we're stuck on the couch and we don't want to get up and do anything. Nothing appeals. We're going nowhere; we've got the Blues.[20]

The term *rajasic* comes from the Sanskrit term *rajas*. Rajas, also one of the three primordial qualities of matter that make up all of creation, is responsible for activity. So rajasic depression is the type of depression where agitation and anxiety predominate. People with rajasic depression may have racing minds and relentless insomnia. Their bodies may be stiff and they may be physically restless, with darting eyes and fingers that won't stay still. Some report difficulties with exhaling fully, a symptom often associated with anxiety. Dr. Somerstein describes it this way:

> A second kind of depression is a fiery, over-energized state that needs calming. We want a lot, but our desires are burning and inchoate, leading everywhere and nowhere.[21]

Although these types of depression seem very different, they share "depressed" sensations of hopelessness and despair. My guess is that this stems from feeling trapped or stuck. Feeling stuck was certainly how I felt during the period when I experienced this kind of depression—which I describe in the preface—because I couldn't find a good way out of my situation. And when you're feeling stuck it's hard to have hope that things can improve.

This part of the chapter will address both types of depression, providing suggestions for each that can help uplift you emotionally, calm you, or both, which may enable you to think more clearly about what to do next and maybe even feel more hopeful. In the yoga tradition, because of the differences between the two types of depression, the positive interventions for the two types differ in significant ways.

Because people with tamasic depression tend to feel lethargic, they typically need physical energizing as well as emotional uplifting. That's why active poses, such as standing poses, backbends, and sequences where you move with your breath are all helpful for tamasic depression. However, people with tamasic depression also suffer from stress, so they may need to include relaxation in their practice

On the other hand, because people with rajasic depression tend to feel agitated, they typically need calming and soothing, rather than energizing. That's why inverted poses, passive backbends and restorative poses are helpful for rajasic depression. However, people with rajasic depression may need to release the physical tension in their bodies first before they are ready to relax, so they may need to include some active poses at the beginning of their practice.

Both forms of depression, however, can be caused by or worsened by stress. After all, depression is a form "freezing" caused by your fight-flight-or-freeze response. Practicing yoga for stress management can reduce your baseline stress levels, which could relieve the depression and/or prevent it from reoccurring. This is why I think it's so important for those of you who are feeling depressed to include stress management practices in every practice you do, even if you don't think you are feeling "stressed." And if you don't yet practice yoga regularly, consider starting to do so, perhaps at least three days a week.

The following sections address positive interventions for the two different types of depression individually.

POSITIVE INTERVENTIONS FOR TAMASIC DEPRESSION

When you're experiencing tamasic depression, you can use yoga to uplift yourself emotionally and energize yourself physically. Chest-opening poses are particularly helpful for both uplifting and energizing you because they encourage taking deeper breaths as you counteract the forward rounding of a "depressed" posture. And although I don't have an explanation for it, many of us have noticed these poses can sometimes just make you feel happier. The chest-opening poses include backbends, both active and passive, as well as poses that stretch the front of your upper chest, such as poses where you take your arms overhead or out to the sides.

Working with your breath can also be energizing and uplifting. You can move in and out of poses with your breath and/or consciously take deeper inhalations.

In addition, because tamasic depression can be caused by or worsened by stress, regularly practicing yoga for stress management can be very helpful over the long term because it can help you stay calmer overall and reduce your baseline stress levels. So that's why I think it's important in your regular practice to incorporate some of your favorite stress management practices into every sequence that you do.

Often people who are experiencing tamasic energy find it hard to start moving. So starting your practice with supported poses that open the chest or with gentle movement is a good strategy. For example, when I feel this way, I like to begin with a passive backbend and Cat-Cow pose. These gentler practices may energize you enough so you feel ready for more active poses. If not, any practice is better than none. Either way, it's a good idea for you to end your practice with a stress-reducing pose, such as a supported inverted pose.

Finally, try to keep your practice short and simple to start. Practice easy and familiar poses, and aim for practicing for a realistic amount of time. That way, it's more likely you'll actually practice than become discouraged. If you're in the middle of a sequence and suddenly feel like you want to do more than you initially planned, you can always add in more poses.

In general, poses and practices that people who are experiencing tamasic depression find helpful include:

1. Standing poses. Because these poses all include an element of balance, they are good for engaging your mind and providing a break from depressing thoughts, and because they are upright, they are stimulating for those who are experiencing lethargy. And many of these poses have arms overhead or out to the side, which helps to open the chest, which invites in deeper inhalations.
2. Backbends. Active backbends are particularly energizing and uplifting, so they can really change your mood. However, they do take some energy just to get into. If you're not feeling ready for them, start with passive backbends to warm up, or simply practice the passive backbends if that's all you can do.
3. Upper chest and shoulder opening. To open your chest, you can do reclined stretches, such as Reclined Arms Overhead pose or a Reclined Twist with your arms

to the sides; you can do shoulder stretches in a seated position, such as Cow-Face pose (Gomukasana); and you can do standing stretches, such as Arms Overhead pose, Standing Cow-Face pose, and Standing Locust pose (Salabhasana).

4. **Moving with your breath.** Moving with your breath is stimulating because it encourages taking deeper breaths. And because you coordinate breath with movement, practicing this way engages your mind in your physical activity, which provides respite from depressing thoughts. You don't have to do a full Sun Salutation to experience these benefits. Even just moving in and out of two poses or in and out of a single pose can have the same effects, such as moving in and out of Bridge pose.

5. **Supported inverted poses.** If you like supported inverted poses, they can be especially beneficial for the stress management part of your practice because they don't require the concentration that other types of relaxation do. Three poses in particular combine a gentle backbend and chest opening with an inverted position: Supported Bridge pose, Supported Legs Up the Wall pose, with arms out to the sides or in a cactus position, and Easy Inverted pose (Ardha Viparita Karani), with arms out to the sides.

6. **Open your eyes.** Try keeping your eyes open in all your poses, even those usually practiced with eyes closed, such as restorative poses and supported inverted poses. And in standing poses, try gazing upward. This may prevent you from turning inward and can bring light into the darkness within you.

7. **Focus on your hands.** In all poses where it is appropriate, try spreading your fingers to move your focus into your hands. Moving your awareness from the center of your body out to your fingertips can expand your sense of self into the outer world.

8. **Focus on your inhalation.** According to Dr. Timothy McCall, people with tamasic depression have shallow breathing and a hard time inhaling. Lengthening your inhalations, either by intentionally taking long, deep inhalations or by practicing a stimulating breath practice, can help uplift you emotionally and energize you physically. (See chapter 7 for information about stimulating breath practices.)

Here are some poses and practices you should consider avoiding when you're experiencing tamasic depression:

1. **Overly challenging poses.** Facing difficulty can be depressing, and poses that feel unsafe can be stressful, so save poses that you struggle with for another time. Lynn Somerstein says it's also a good idea to avoid poses that feel unnecessarily stressful for your body until you're feeling better.

2. **Poses that cause brooding.** Poses where you turn inward, such as forward bends, or restorative poses where you feel like you are being left alone with your thoughts, can cause you to spiral downward, increasing your depression. If that's how any pose makes you feel, skip it for now.

3. **Meditation.** Although meditation is considered to be "calming," if you're feeling depressed, sitting alone with your thoughts could cause a downward spiral. Lynn Somerstein says it can lead to "endless recriminatory ruminations" making you feel worse. She recommends avoiding the practice in these circumstances.

RESPONDING IN THE MOMENT TO TAMASIC DEPRESSION

Although tamasic depression doesn't come on as suddenly as anger or anxiety, if you notice yourself starting to spiral downward into feelings of depression, there are many different yoga techniques you can use to quickly uplift yourself emotionally and energize yourself physically. And many are poses you can do in everyday clothes. Experiment with the various options listed below to see which ones you find helpful. And if it feels comfortable, you can use any of these moments as an opportunity to take a "precious pause" and consider what a skillful response to the situation would be for you (see Listening and Responding to Painful Emotions on page 137).

1. **Bridge pose.** B. K. S. Iyengar says that for depression, if you have time for just one pose, Bridge pose is the best choice. This pose opens your chest, inviting in deeper breaths, but at the same time it is a partial inversion, which is quieting for your mind and nervous system. Depending on whether you want to focus more on stimulation or calming, there are three different ways to practice Bridge pose: with support, as an active backbend, and as a vinyasa. I find the version with support very calming and the vinyasa version very emotionally uplifting. For the vinyasa, practice for 6 to 12 rounds.

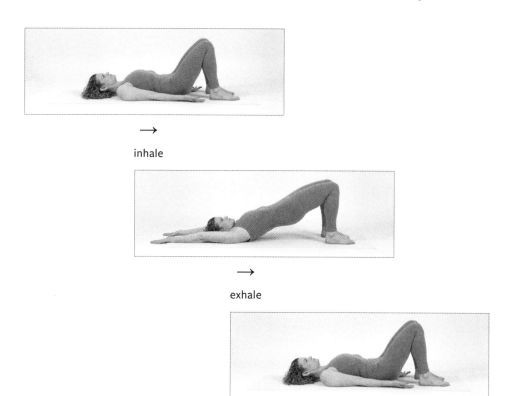

→

inhale

→

exhale

2. **Arms Overhead vinyasa.** Moving with your breath is energizing, and taking your arms above your head can be emotionally uplifting. When you raise your arms overhead on your inhalation, extend your fingers and gaze up toward them, reaching upward with both your body and your mind.

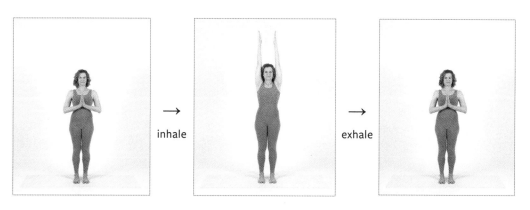

→

inhale

→

exhale

3. Cat-Cow pose. This gentle vinyasa a good way to begin moving and breathing consciously. You can use it to bring yourself into your body in the moment or, if you have time for more than one pose, as a way to get started a when energy levels and motivation are low. Practice for 3 to 12 rounds.

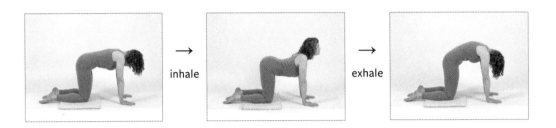

inhale   exhale

4. Warrior 2 pose arms. This simple pose opens your chest, inviting in deeper breaths, and allows you to move your awareness away from your center out to the external world. Starting in Mountain pose, on an inhalation sweep your arms out to the side. Open your chest, lengthen your arms outward, and extend out through your fingertips. As you look straight ahead, imagine your mind's gaze is traveling outward to your fingertips. Continue for a minute or two, breathing naturally, and then exhale and release. Stand quietly for a moment, keeping your chest open, and notice how you feel.

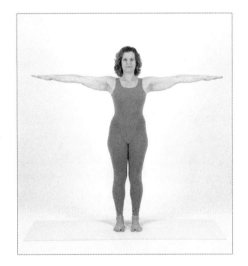

5. Standing Locust pose. This simple standing backbend opens your chest to invite in a deeper breath and releases tight muscles in your front body. As you practice, focus on taking deep breaths, especially deep, full inhalations. Practice for 30 to 90 seconds.

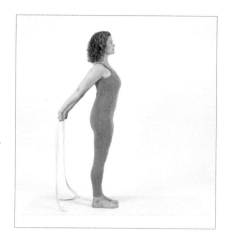

6. Supported Backbend. If you're very low on energy and lying down is the only thing that feels possible, a simple Supported Backbend (Salamba Urdva Dhanurasana) is a good way to open your chest and invite in deeper breaths. Practice for 3 to 10 minutes.

Because the reclined poses where you use a support under your head and torso—including Supported Reclined Crossed Legs (Salamba Supta Sukasana) or Reclined Cobbler's poses, and Supported Savasana—all create a gentle, supported backbend, those are good alternatives as well.

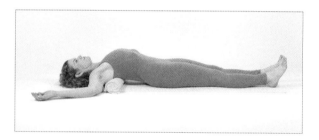

7. Focus on your inhalation. It can be helpful in the moment just to focus on inhaling completely. For a few minutes, make every inhalation full, complete, and nourishing. As Patricia Walden says about using this practice for tamasic depression, "What comes with that is a feeling of life returning, a feeling of warmth that percolates throughout your chest at the beginning, but then throughout your entire body."[22]

Of course, if any of the coping mechanisms in chapter 2 are helpful in these circumstances, those are also good options for you. If you have more time in the moment, you can do a longer practice, such as the Active Uplifting Practice.

MOVING THROUGH TAMASIC DEPRESSION

When you experience tamasic depression, you will probably feel lethargic and unmotivated. So in addition to needing some emotional uplifting, you will also need physical energizing. Standing poses, backbends, and sequences where you move with your breath are all helpful for tamasic depression because they are both uplifting and energizing, but they take some effort. So if you're feeling unmotivated, starting your practice with something easy and simple that is mildly energizing can prepare you for more demanding poses. That's why the Active Uplifting Practice on page 127 starts with a supported backbend and Cat-Cow pose before the more active backbends. You'll then be ready to move into the more active poses.

For the active part of your practice, you can practice whichever poses you prefer, though in general backbend shapes, such as Warrior 1, may be more helpful than forward-bend shapes, such as Standing Forward Bend or Pyramid pose (Parsvottanasana). If staying in a single pose for too long makes you depressed, it's fine to practice shorter holds, or you can stick with poses or sequences where you move in and out of poses with your breath.

Because stress can cause or worsen tamasic depression, it's a good idea to end every sequence with one or more of your favorite stress management practices. In the Active Uplifting Practice, I'm suggesting Savasana with legs on a chair as your relaxation pose. That's because it's a good counter-pose for backbends as well as a good relaxation pose. But you can practice anything in chapter 3 that works for you as the stress management component of your practice. For restorative poses, choose backbend shapes, such as Reclined Cobbler's pose, which can be emotionally uplifting, rather than forward-bend shapes. In Savasana, try a supported version, with your torso lifted and your chest open, rather than lying flat.

After practicing this way, if you're ready to "listen" to the signals your feelings of depression are sending you and to consider skillful responses, see Listening and Responding to Painful Emotions on page 137 for more information.

Active Uplifting Practice

For this practice, focus on your inhalation, making it full, complete, and nourishing. If you want to practice longer, you can include mini Sun Salutations as shown in the Moving Through Grief Practice in chapter 5 or standing poses such as Warrior 1, 2, and 3, after the Dropped-Knee Lunge pose (Vanarasana). For the Locust (Salabhasana) and Bow poses (Dhanurasana), repeat them twice, resting in Prone Savasana in between. For Bridge pose, rest in the starting position between repetitions.

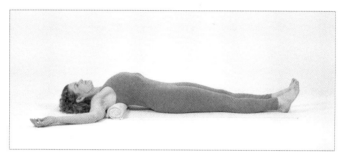

1. Supported Backbend, *1 to 3 minutes*

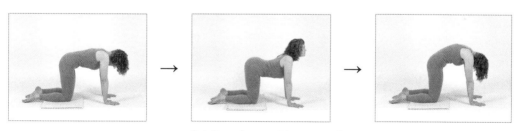

2. Cat-Cow vinyasa, *6 to 12 rounds*

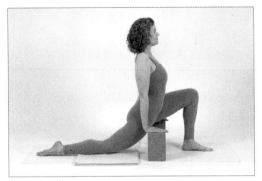

3. Dropped-Knee Lunge pose,
   30 to 90 seconds per side

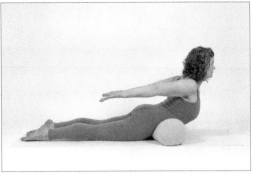

4. Supported Locust pose,
   30 to 60 seconds, twice

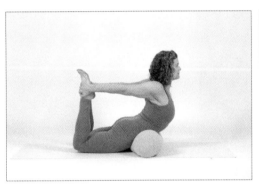

5. Supported Bow, *30 to 60 seconds, twice*

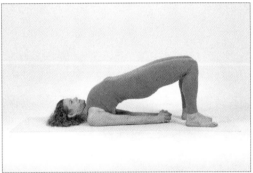

6. Bridge pose, *30 to 60 seconds, twice*

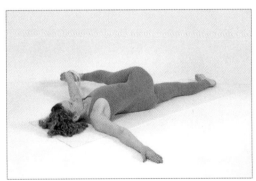

7. Reclined Twist, *30 to 90 seconds per side*

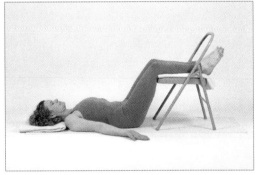

8. Savasana with chair, *3 to 10 minutes*

POSITIVE INTERVENTIONS FOR RAJASIC DEPRESSION

When you're experiencing rajasic depression, you can use yoga to calm down from your agitation and also to uplift yourself emotionally. Because rajasic depression has so much in common with anxiety, such as a racing mind, physical restlessness, insomnia, and digestive problems, any of the anxiety practices or sequences described under Fear and Anxiety on page 102, if they work for you, can be helpful when you're experiencing rajasic depression as well. But for rajasic depression you can also counteract your feelings of depression by practicing chest-opening poses for their uplifting qualities. These poses may uplift you emotionally because they encourage taking deeper breaths as you counteract the forward rounding of a "depressed" posture. And although I don't have an explanation for it, many of us have noticed these poses can sometimes just make you feel happier. The chest-opening poses for rajasic depression include passive backbends as well as poses that stretch the front of your upper chest, such as poses where you take your arms overhead or out to the sides.

Finally, try to keep your practice short and simple to start. Practice easy and familiar poses, and aim for a realistic amount of time. That way, it's more likely you'll actually practice than become discouraged. If you're in the middle of a sequence and suddenly feel like you want to do more than you initially planned, you can always add in more poses.

In general, poses and practices that people who are experiencing rajasic depression find helpful include:

1. **Standing poses:** These are helpful for burning off your excess energy, preparing you for quieter practices. Many also have arms overhead or out to the sides, which can release the tightness in your chest and improve your exhalations. And because these poses all include an element of balance, they are also good for engaging your mind, providing a break from anxious or depressing thoughts.

2. **Upper chest and shoulder opening.** To release the tightness in your chest and improve your exhalations, you can do reclined stretches, such as Reclined Arms Overhead pose or a Reclined Twist with your arms to the sides; you can do shoulder stretches in a seated position, such as Cow-Face pose; and you can do standing stretches, such as Arms Overhead pose, Standing Cow-Face pose, and Standing Locust pose. To choose which kind, keep in mind that reclined stretches are the most relaxing, and the standing stretches are the most stimulating.

3. **Moving slowly with your breath.** Because you coordinate breath with movement, moving in and out of poses with your breath engages your mind in your physical activity, giving you some respite from anxious or depressed thoughts, and it can also improve your breathing. Slow vinyasas can also help burn off excess energy. You can do a longer vinyasa, such as a Sun Salutation, or you can just move in and out of two poses or in and out of one pose. Just be sure to keep it slow because moving too quickly—and breathing too quickly—can be overstimulating.

4. **Supported backbends.** Active backbends are very energizing and can be too stimulating for those experiencing rajasic depression. So turn to supported backbends for their uplifting qualities and to improve your breathing. You can practice a simple supported backbend like the one shown in the Calming Uplifting Practice on page 135 or any other supported backbends you're familiar with. In the Iyengar tradition, there is a whole range of supported backbends that you can do with a chair.

5. **Supported inverted poses.** If you like supported inverted poses, those can be especially beneficial for the stress management part of your practice because they don't require the concentration that other types of "relaxation" do and can be easier to practice when you're feeling agitated. Three poses in particular combine a gentle backbend and chest opening with an inverted position: Supported Bridge pose; Supported Legs Up the Wall pose, with arms out to the sides or in a cactus position; and Easy Inverted pose, with arms out to the sides.

6. **Open your eyes.** Try keeping your eyes open in all your poses, even those usually practiced with eyes closed, such as restorative poses and supported inverted poses. And in standing poses, try looking upward. This may prevent you from turning inward and can bring light into the dark space within you.

7. **Focus on your hands.** In all poses where it is appropriate, try spreading your fingers to move your focus into your hands. Moving your awareness from the center of your body out to your fingertips can expand your sense of self into the outer world.

8. **Focus on your exhalation.** According to Dr. McCall, people with rajasic depression tend to breathe quickly and erratically, and they find it hard to exhale completely. Lengthening your exhalations, either by intentionally making your exhalations longer or by practicing a calming breath practice can help improve your breathing and quiet you down.

Here are some poses and practices you should consider avoiding when you're experiencing rajasic depression:

1. **Relaxing poses that aren't relaxing.** If you feel restless and agitated in any pose that is supposedly relaxing, such as a restorative pose, try another form of relaxation that works better for you or do some active poses or other physical activity first, such as taking a long walk, and then try relaxing after that.
2. **Poses that cause brooding.** Although forward bends can be calming for those with rajasic depression, for some they can cause you to turn inward and ruminate. If you find that these or any poses cause you to become more depressed, try something else instead.
3. **Overly stimulating poses.** While it's good to tire yourself out when you're experiencing rajasic depression, active backbends, jumping from pose to pose, and moving quickly with your breath could fire up your agitation or anxiety. Consider avoiding these practices until you're feeling more grounded.
5. **Stimulating breath practices.** Not all pranayama is calming, and some forms actually stimulate your nervous system, which could increase your anxiety or agitation. (See Breath Practices for Self-Regulation on page 191 for information.)
4. **Meditation.** Although meditation is considered to be "calming," if you're feeling depressed, sitting alone with your thoughts could cause a downward spiral into deeper depression. Dr. Somerstein says it can lead to "endless recriminatory ruminations" making you feel worse. She recommends avoiding the practice in these circumstances.

RESPONDING IN THE MOMENT TO RAJASIC DEPRESSION

Although you probably won't feel a sudden burst of rajasic depression the way you might feel a sudden burst of anger, you may feel a surge of anxiety that could lead to rajasic depression. In this case, it's good to take action to reduce your anxiety. Because I had a very bad experience with rajasic depression myself many years ago, whenever I start to feel anxious, I practice Supported Legs Up the Wall pose as soon as possible.

Any of the suggestions for anxiety under Responding in the Moment to Fear or Anxiety on page 107 could be very helpful to calm you down in times like these. But you also might want to experiment with some positive interventions that are listed below, which are both calming and emotionally uplifting. And if it feels comfortable, you can use any of these moments as an opportunity to take a "precious pause" and consider what a skillful response to the situation would be for you (see Listening and Responding to Painful Emotions on page 137).

1. **Supported Legs Up the Wall pose.** This pose, which combines a slight backbend with an inverted pose, can provide both chest opening and powerful stress reduction. Take your arms either out to the sides or in a cactus position. You can also get similar effects with Easy Inverted pose with your arms out to your sides. Practice for 5 to 20 minutes.

2. **Supported Bridge pose.** This is B. K. S. Iyengar's go-to pose for depression because it opens the chest, allowing deeper breathing, and at the same time it is quieting for the mind. For rajasic depression, practicing with support enhances the calming aspect of the pose. There are many different versions of Supported Bridge pose, including with bent knees and also with straight legs. Here's a nice version with straight legs you could try in addition to the bent-knee version shown in the Calming Uplifting Practice on page 135. You can either use two bolsters or a bolster over a blanket stack. Make sure both your head and your shoulders are touching the floor! Practice for 3 to 10 minutes.

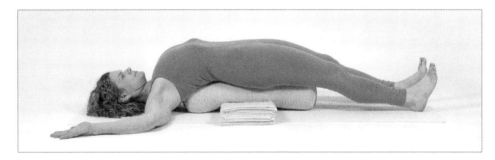

3. **Supported Backbend.** For some of the emotionally uplifting quality of a backbend without the stimulation, you can practice any supported backbend you like. In addition to the simple one with a rolled blanket shown in the Calming Uplifting Practice, here's a version I like to practice using two blocks, with one at its lowest height and the other at its medium height. Practice for 2 to 5 minutes.

Because the reclined poses where you use a support under your head and torso—including Supported Reclined Crossed Legs or Supported Reclined Cobbler's pose and Supported Savasana—all create a gentle, supported backbend, those are good alternatives as well.

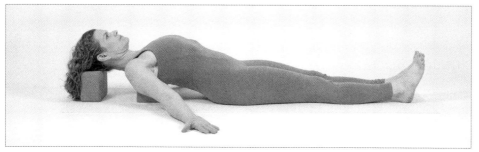

4. **Focus on your exhalation.** It can be helpful in the moment just to focus on exhaling completely. For a few minutes, make every exhalation long and smooth, imagining each exhalation relaxes your chest muscles. As Patricia Walden says about this practice for rajasic depression, "What comes with the space inside your chest is also space in your mental body. You're not holding anymore."[23] Dr. Somerstein suggests blowing out your breath through an open mouth while making a sound.

Of course, if any of the coping skills in chapter 2 are helpful in these circumstances, those are also good options for you. If you have more time in the moment, you can do a longer practice, such as the Calming Uplifting Practice or either of the sequences for anxiety that are shown earlier in this chapter.

MOVING THROUGH RAJASIC DEPRESSION

When you experience rajasic depression, you will probably feel hyper and agitated as well as depressed. This means that in addition to needing some emotional uplifting, you will also need calming. However, people who are experiencing rajasic depression often find it hard to start with quieter practices. So practicing active poses first, including standing poses and/or slower vinyasas, is a good way to burn off your excess energy. That's why the Calming Uplifting Practice starts with several standing poses. If staying in a single pose for too long makes you agitated, it's fine to practice shorter holds.

After burning off excess energy, you will then be ready to move on to quieter poses. At this point you can either practice supported backbends for their uplifting qualities or go directly to stress reducing poses or practices for their calming qualities.

If you want to do both, practice the backbends before the stress management poses. Although supported backbends aren't as stimulating as active ones, because they open your chest and improve your breathing—your inhalations as well as your exhalations—they still might be slightly stimulating. But it's worth trying them to see if their uplifting quality is helpful for you.

Because stress can cause or worsen rajasic depression, I suggest that you end every sequence with one or more of your favorite stress management practices. In the Calming Uplifting Practice, I'm suggesting Easy Inverted pose or Supported Legs Up the Wall pose as your relaxation pose. That's because supported inverted poses can be very helpful for those experiencing rajasic depression. But you can practice anything in chapter 3 that works for you for the stress management component of your practice. For restorative poses, choose backbend shapes, such as Reclined Cobbler's pose, which can be emotionally uplifting, rather than forward-bend shapes. In Savasana, try a supported version, with your torso lifted and your chest open, rather than lying flat.

After practicing this way, if you're ready to "listen" to the signals your feelings of depression are sending you and to consider skillful responses, see Listening and Responding to Painful Emotions on page 137 for more information.

Calming Uplifting Practice

For this practice, in the active poses focus on your hands by spreading your fingers. In the last three poses, focus on your exhalations, making them long and complete. If you want to lengthen the practice, start with the mini Sun Salutation shown in the Moving Through Grief Practice in chapter 5 or add in more standing poses after the Warrior 3 pose (Virabhadrasana 3).

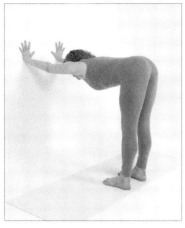

1. Half Downward-Facing Dog pose, *30 to 60 seconds*

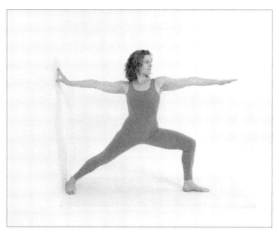

2. Warrior 2 pose, *30 to 60 seconds per side*

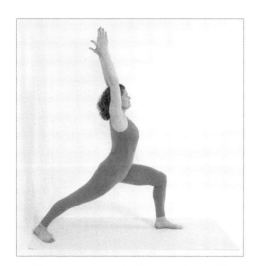

3. Warrior 1 pose, *30 to 60 seconds per side*

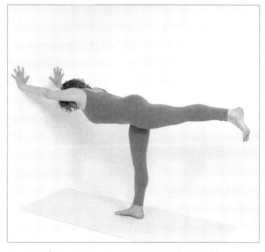

4. Warrior 3 pose, *30 to 60 seconds per side*

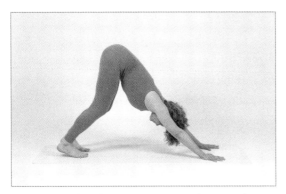

5. Downward-Facing Dog pose, *30 to 60 seconds*

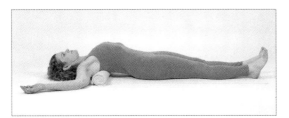

6. Supported Backbend, *3 to 5 minutes*

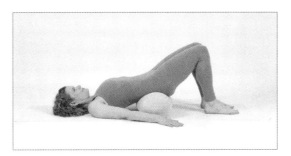

7. Supported Bridge pose, *3 to 10 minutes*

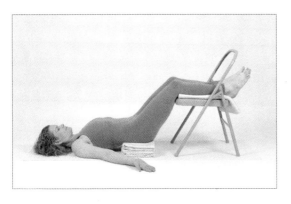

8. Easy Inverted pose or Supported Legs Up the Wall pose, *5 to 20 minutes*

Listening and Responding to Painful Emotions

Awareness and acceptance of the emotions is the first step towards dealing with them. Sit with them quietly and let them stew and see what stories might come up. These stories are yours to accept and perhaps modify for the future. Consider changing the plot.

—Dr. Lynn Somerstein, "Anger and Yoga: An Interview with
Dr. Lynn Somerstein," *Yoga for Healthy Aging Blog*

Before you can respond skillfully to a painful emotion, you may need to set aside some time to listen for the signals it is sending you. When you feel up to it, there are four basic ways to tune in to those signals: pausing briefly, practicing mindfulness meditation to study the emotion, practicing self-inquiry to study the emotion, and observing the emotion as you practice yoga poses. Practicing mindfulness meditation to study an intense emotion is described under How to Practice Mindfulness Meditation in chapter 7, and self-inquiry is discussed under Practicing Self-Inquiry in chapter 8. This section covers pausing briefly and using your asana practice to study emotions.

Which way you choose to do your "listening" depends on how much time you have and what you feel comfortable with. Just don't do anything that makes you feel worse.

PAUSING BRIEFLY TO LISTEN

In the brief moment between when you experience a strong emotion and then react to it, you have the opportunity to pause briefly. For both yoga practitioners and for Buddhists, this moment is considered so important for responding skillfully to thoughts and emotions that it is called a "sacred "or "precious" pause. Jack Kornfield said,

> In a moment of stopping, we break the spell between past result and automatic reaction. When we pause, we can notice the actual experience, the pain or pleasure, fear or excitement. In the stillness before our habits arise, we become free.[24]

To take the precious pause, you step back and observe what you're feeling—along with any associated physical symptoms—without reacting to them.

As I discussed earlier in the chapter, taking this precious pause when you feel anger, fear, or anxiety surging may reduce the intensity of the emotion itself. At this time, you also have the opportunity to listen for signals the emotion might be sending you. Perhaps you or someone else is in actual danger and should respond by taking protective or evasive actions. Having lived through a serious earthquake, I feel a surge of fear every time my house starts shaking. I listen to my fear by pausing to assess what is really happening. Sometimes there really is an earthquake, and if I think it's serious enough I'll take shelter.

But you can also notice if an emotional response is automatic, based on previous experiences you have had. Dr. Lauzé says that that our amygdala, which triggers the fight-flight-or-freeze response—and the intense emotions associated with it—is not very sophisticated and has "little ability to calculate the appropriateness" of triggering your nervous system this way. That's why reacting immediately isn't always the best response. Because of my previous experience with a serious earthquake, my fear is triggered every time the house starts to shake, but frequently it turns out that it is the just washing machine below me that's causing the house to shake.

Pausing regularly this way not only allows you to really listen to strong emotional reactions you're having but it builds a habit that you can use throughout your day to respond more skillfully to whatever situations you face.

PRACTICING YOGA POSES TO LISTEN

By listening to my inner voice without judgment, I felt a lot lighter. Before that, I didn't even know someone inside of me was speaking to me.

—Yoriko Matsumoto, Yoga for Depression teacher

Some of you may find it easier to observe emotions when you are moving and engaged with your body as well as your mind. To do this, when you practice your yoga poses, allow yourself to notice whatever emotions come up during your practice as well as the physical sensations that are associated with them. As always, listening in your yoga practice means observing without reacting or making judgments. Yoriko Matsumoto found her asana practice was the easiest way to listen to her depression, saying "Your body and muscles feed your brain back a lot of information. It is so difficult to listen to your heart, but if it's your body it's easier because you feel it."[25]

You can either just practice any type of sequence you want or you can intention-ally practice poses that provoke an emotional reaction, such as poses you're afraid of or that you strongly dislike for whatever reason. Then, in a safe environment—when you're by yourself and can stop at any time—you observe your emotional reactions to the poses. I learned a lot from watching fear arise in certain types of poses.

RESPONDING SKILLFULLY TO PAINFUL EMOTIONS

When we give our bodies time to relax and engage in activities grounded in the pres-ent moment, we also grow the ability to put a little space between a triggering, or fear-inducing event and our response to it. This space between a trigger and an au-tomatic response gives us enough time to think about and choose a skillful response, rather than react impulsively or automatically.

—Dr. Scott Lauzé

For almost all situations, keeping the yamas in mind can help you respond with skill to whatever you are facing. The yamas are yoga's guiding principles for how to conduct yourself in all your relationships, within your community, and with the world at large. Adopting these principles can help you live with greater equanimity and may provide a structure that helps you make decisions.

The list of specific yamas varies from one yoga tradition to another, but virtually all include nonviolence (*ahimsa*) as the most important yama. According to Edwin Bryant ahimsa is the "root" of all the other yamas and "the goal of the other *yamas* is to achieve *ahimsa* and enhance it."[26]

The ancient yogis observed that one of our main problems as a species is a tendency not only toward taking violent actions but also having violent thoughts about other people. And taking violent actions and having violent thoughts not only interfere with your peace of mind but also cause violent relationships, which perpetuate the violence in your life and in your community. These ideas had a profound influence on Mohandas K. Gandhi, who was himself a serious practitioner of yoga, and led to his successful non-violent form of social activism, which secured the independence of India. This in turn directly inspired the nonviolent activism of Martin Luther King Jr. and Nelson Mandela.

In our personal lives, practicing nonviolence as we respond to others can im-prove our relationships as well as help foster peace within us because there will be less "drama" in our life and fewer upsetting thoughts and emotions running through our mind. Cultivating Universal Kindness in chapter 8 discusses how you can intentionally cultivate nonviolence in your relationships, in your community, and toward yourself with the four practices of universal kindness.

Keep in mind, however, that practicing nonviolence also means refraining from harming yourself. So, if a situation is dangerous for you and there is no workable or healthy solution, the skillful response could be to walk away.

In addition to the yama nonviolence (ahimsa), yoga teachers in the West focus mostly on the four other yamas listed in Patanjali's Yoga Sutras. Each of them can help to reduce conflicts in your relationships and foster more contentment in your life. Briefly, they are:

1. Truthfulness (*satya*): Practicing honesty in action, speech, and thought.
2. Non-stealing (*asteya*): Refraining from taking things that belong to others, including both material things and ideas (such as taking credit for someone else's work).
3. Non-possessiveness (*aparigraha*): Limiting your possessions to only what is necessary and not wishing for more than you have. And because this yama also means "non-holding," it also means not clinging to thoughts and emotions that cloud your judgment and disturb your equanimity. Let them go rather than allowing them to become obsessions.
4. Sexual restraint (*brahmacarya*): While this originally meant "chastity," or refraining from sex completely, for us ordinary householders in modern times we can think of this yama as sexual responsibility. Exactly how you interpret that is up to you.

Chapter 8 introduces some additional yamas from other yoga texts and provides suggestions for how to put the yamas into practice. All of these yamas can help reduce the "drama" in your life and help you respond skillfully to whatever situations you are facing. But of all the yamas, nonviolence takes precedence. For example, if you're angry and want to speak the truth, responding skillfully would mean finding a way of expressing that truth that is also nonviolent—or even keeping silent if necessary.

Even as you keep the yamas in mind, however, the skillful way to respond to an emotion can also depend on why the emotion was triggered. After all, as I said earlier, we're often triggered inappropriately! So when anger, fear, or depression is triggered due to patterns of behavior created by previous experiences, the automatic response you feel, while natural, might be clouding the issues for you, preventing you from finding a new way of navigating the situation. In that case, a skillful response might mean taking a different tack, such as cultivating compassion (*karuna*) for all those involved in a conflict (see Cultivating Compassion (*Karuna*) on page 247).

And when you realize that resentment, fear, or any other emotion has been festering within you, working on letting that go might be the best solution. There are many different yoga techniques that you can use to release your painful emotion so you can move on. For example, you can let go of the anger by practicing detachment, and you can dissolve anger, fear, or other painful emotions by cultivating loving-kindness, compassion, sympathetic joy, equanimity, or forgiveness.

After using her asana practice and other methods to "dissipate" some of her anger, Charissa Loftis started practicing compassion for herself. This led her to be able to cultivate compassion for her parents, especially for her father who was a Vietnam War veteran. She says this helped "dissolve" her anger, creating an opening for her to see her family situation from a new perspective and to change her actions accordingly, leading to a positive outcome for the entire family. And to recover from a traumatic experience, my colleague Ram Rao and his wife, Padma, found that practicing forgiveness (*kshama*) helped them to "free ourselves from the traumatic past and move on with those events cleared from our lives."

Letting Go in chapter 8 covers in depth how to let go of thoughts and emotions that are not serving you, including by cultivating compassion and forgiveness.

5

Moving Through Grief

Proceed with your whole heart into the practice that calls to
you. Do not avoid your grief, sorrow will come and your heart
will open to find space for joyfulness sometimes, too.
—Dr. Lynn Somerstein, "Grief and Yoga: An Interview with
Dr. Lynn Somerstein," *Yoga for Healthy Aging Blog*

Although we typically associate feelings of grief with the death of a loved one, grief
can be a response to any significant loss or change, such as the diagnosis of a chronic
disease, the loss of a home, or the end of an important relationship. For example, Erin
Collins, who is a yoga teacher, hospice nurse, and end-of-life doula, says that during
her twenty-five years of practicing yoga, grief had "visited her door" many times. In her
twenties, along with grieving the death of her grandmother, she grieved the end of her
long-term love relationship as well the end of the plans they'd made to sail around the
world together, an adventure she'd long been dreaming of.

Bonnie Maeda, a hospice nurse and yoga therapist, says that we are always going
through changes, and some are easier to accept than others. Sometimes you may even
be surprised to realize that what you are feeling after a loss is actually grief.

In addition to feeling grief over personal losses, we may also feel collective grief over
events that cause the suffering of people within our community, our country, or even

across the world, whether from natural disasters, racial persecution, food shortages, or political oppression. The degree of grief you feel for these different types of losses will vary. But recognizing that you're grieving and accepting the way you're feeling without judgment is as important for any type of loss as it is for grieving the death of a loved one. I vividly remember a short-lived bout of grief I experienced the first day I dropped my younger child off at our local public middle school. Knowing what my older child and her friends had been through during their middle school years, my heart broke imagining what might lie in store for the children of that school lining up for classes that day. Before this is over, I thought, someone would be bullied, someone would be pregnant, someone would be taking drugs, someone would be assaulted, and I broke down in tears.

It's also important to recognize that grief is a very complex emotion—or maybe a set of emotions. Even though there are many stereotypes about what grief is, in real life people seem to respond to loss, even great loss, very differently from one another. For example, Beth Gibbs said that when her husband died, "I was mad, I was sad, I was exhausted, but I wasn't depressed." On the other hand, Bonnie Maeda described her grief over the death of her youngest son, who was murdered, this way: "The hole I fell into was so deep and so dark I did not know if I would ever recover."

Because her yoga practice was an integral part of her healing—which she describes as a slow climb out of the "dark hole"—Bonnie now teaches yoga for grief. She has helped me to understand that there is no right way or wrong way to grieve. In an interview I did with her, she put it this way:

> The grief process varies from person to person as well as from one type of loss to another. I believe what is important is to be aware of what your individual reaction and process is to a given loss or significant change. There is no right or wrong.[1]

That's why I feel it's important to keep in mind—both for yourself and others whom you want to support while they are grieving—that how each person experiences grief will be different. And the way people grieve may also vary with the individual circumstances of a particular loss, not to mention your particular personality, your stage in life, and how much experience you have with loss.

After my mother died—a death that was expected—I was very surprised at how I felt in the immediate aftermath. I had imagined that I would experience intense feelings of sorrow and loss, but instead when the time came, I kept saying to myself, "Why does grief feel so much like stress?" Recognizing that I felt stressed, however, allowed me to choose the right practices for me. As I practiced very long sessions of Legs Up the Wall pose, my go-to pose for stress, and I began to calm down, the tears came. So a good place to start practicing yoga for grief is to accept whatever you are feeling without judgment. You'll then be able to find ways to support yourself through your grieving process, to take actions when you feel stuck, and give yourself a break when needed.

GRIEF NEEDS TO RUN ITS COURSE

Each person, each loss, each significant change has its own unique course. There is no simple recipe or one way to process grief.

—Bonnie Maeda, "Grief and Yoga: An Interview with Bonnie Maeda, RN,"
Yoga for Healthy Aging Blog

Although the way we experience grief varies from person to person and from situation to situation, one thing all the grief experts I consulted with agreed on was that grief needs to be fully felt. Erin Collins said that it took her time to understand this because in her twenties she thought of grief as something to "escape" rather than as something to be "experienced." It was only later when she practiced yoga through two losses, the end of her long-term love relationship and the death of a dear friend who died tragically in an avalanche—something that left her feeling overcome with depression and grief—that she realized: "We turn to yoga not to escape our lives, but to more fully experience them."[2] Of course, allowing yourself to fully experience grief may be challenging. Dr. Lynn Somerstein even says, "Mourning calls for courage." But grief experts say that the pain of grief won't diminish until it is heard and acknowledged. So pushing your feelings away or covering them up can cause you to become stuck and keep you from moving through your grief. Sharon Salzberg says that what has helped her is taking the perspective that grief is an intrinsic part of human experience.

> What has helped me with grieving is just having the perspective that suffering is part of life, and that it's not a separation of life, and that our practices in our communities are intended to allow us to hold suffering as part of our human experience.[3]

And you can make grieving somewhat easier by supporting yourself through the process, as I will describe next. You can also take breaks when you need to. And if you do feel stuck, there are ways to use your yoga practice to help you "move through" your grief.

In addition, grief needs to run its full course, for as long as it takes. In the same way that grief is experienced differently from person to person, the time it takes a person to move through it also varies. So even though we hear may hear "rules" about how long it takes to recover from the end of a marriage or the death of a spouse, or people even say, "You should be over it now," the process of grief should, as Bonnie Maeda says, "be given as much time as it needs." Lynn Somerstein adds, "Grieving is an organic process that needs to run through the body/mind in its own way and its own time, and like a deep yoga practice it affects every cell."[4]

IS GRIEF A SIGNAL?

In chapter 4, I discussed how painful emotions can be important signals that are worth attending to. When you take the time to listen to what a painful emotion is telling you, you can then respond more skillfully to the situation or person that triggered the emotion.

But what message is the emotion of "grief" sending you? I wonder whether it might not simply be that you lost someone or something important. I find it both comforting and beautiful to think that the grief you feel when someone you love has died is—as Christopher D. Wallis says—a form of your love for them: "the intensity of the pain you feel when a loved one passes away is another form of your love for them—experienced in that way, it becomes a thing of sharp beauty."[5] Responding skillfully to grief may mean striving to accept impermanence (see Accepting Impermanence on page 200). However, in other cases, grief over the loss of something important might be a signal that you need to take an action of some kind, for example, to repair a broken relationship or to end a toxic one. For grief over suffering in your community or in another part of the world, this response may spur you to engage in acts of service or even social activism to help provide solutions to root causes.

HOW YOGA HELPS WITH GRIEF

Yoga helps us stay in the moment while realizing that moments are temporary and so are we. We learn to be patient with pain and not jump away from it or from ourselves, to endure, to treasure joy, to know life and all things are fleeting.

—Dr. Lynn Somerstein "Grief and Yoga: An Interview with Dr. Lynn Somerstein,"
Yoga for Healthy Aging Blog

Because yoga includes so many options for helping you move through grief—movement, relaxation, breath practices, meditation, and philosophy—it allows you to create a personalized practice based on your needs, abilities, and preferences. You can either design your practice yourself or ask your yoga teacher to help you design one. Just be willing to experiment because if you think what you're doing is working, it's working. And if you think it's not working, you can just try something else! In this section I'll provide an overview of the basic ways yoga can help, with more specific suggestions and sequences in the sections that follow.

Being present with grief. The first way is that you can use yoga to provide yourself with safe, comfortable, and self-compassionate ways to grieve. Allowing yourself to "witness" your grief in a nonjudgmental way can help you move through your grief and may even reduce the intensity of it. Some grief experts refer to this as "holding space" for grief, a practice they consider to be essential. I'll describe several ways to do this under Being Present with Grief on page 148.

Supporting yourself. You can use your yoga practice to take care of your body, mind, and heart during times of grief. Depending on how you experience grief, many of the techniques I've suggested in chapters 2 through 4 may be very helpful, and I'll discuss why later. And if none of those work for you, the section Supporting Your Body, Mind, and Heart on page 156 has additional options as well as a practice for fatigue.

Moving through grief. When movement is something that you always find helpful, you may be able to encourage your grief to move through you physically by using gentle movements, whether gentle stretches, easy poses of any kind, or moving with your breath. This can be especially helpful when you're feeling stuck. See the section Moving Through Grief on page 160 for more information and a sequence of poses.

Taking a break. A mindful asana practice can provide some temporary respite and may even make you feel lighter afterward. You can just practice some of your favorite yoga poses mindfully as described in chapter 2, but there are also some specific suggestions for what to practice as well as a sequence in Taking a Break from Grief on page 166.

Accepting impermanence. During 2020, the yoga teacher Barrie Risman and I talked about how we both were surprised to find that yoga philosophy sustained us through that difficult year more than any other aspect of our yoga practices. So, if you feel up to it, reading about the yoga philosophy that I cover in chapter 8, turning to your favorite yoga text, or even taking a course on yoga philosophy may provide you with some comfort.

I also have some suggestions for practices you might want to avoid during periods of grief:

1. Avoid engaging in quieter practices if they're not working for you for any reason.
2. Avoid poses or practices that makes you feel unsafe.
3. Approach backbends with caution and see how you respond to them. They can be uplifting, but they may also trigger "deeper" emotions that you're not ready for, especially deeper backbends.

Being Present with Grief

When we allow ourselves to feel our feelings fully and bring compassion to our experiences, this process can lessen the intensity and return us to a sense of well-being.
—Bonnie Maeda, "Grief and Yoga: An Interview with Bonnie Maeda, RN,"
Yoga for Healthy Aging Blog

Traditionally, being present with grief—or "holding space" as it is often called these days—is a form of mindfulness meditation. In this practice, you allow yourself to witness your grief by observing—without judgment and with self-compassion—whatever feelings arise as you sit with your grief. However, if you feel that you're not ready for this type of practice or you would simply prefer to practice being present with your grief in a more structured way, you can use a traditional yoga concentration practice to focus on the person or people you're grieving for.

Obviously, both ways of practicing are things you shouldn't do until you feel ready. When Jivana Heyman's mother died, he waited to return to his regular practice until the time was right for him, and he then found that being present with his grief was more helpful than he had been expecting:

> But, immediately after my mother died, I found myself avoiding my practice. I couldn't bring myself to sit in meditation or do any asanas. I knew that if I sat with my feelings they would come out even more strongly, and I wasn't ready for them. But when I finally got myself back to my practice, I had the opposite experience from what I expected. Instead of feeling like I was going deeper into the sadness, I felt a kind of inner calmness that was so surprising.[6]

When you do start practice, make sure that if your practice ever feels like it's too much for you that you allow yourself to stop. You can then switch to any yoga pose or practice that you find comforting or calming, or simply move on to another activity that you think will be more helpful for you at this time, such as taking a walk or talking with a friend.

And as you practice either way of being present, do your best to be nonjudgmental about the thoughts, emotions, and physical sensations you observe and refrain from making any judgments about how "well" you are doing the practice.

I'll start by discussing how to choose a pose or poses that you can use when you're ready to be present with grief. I'll then discuss the two basic ways you can practice being present.

CHOOSING COMFORTABLE POSES

Being present with your grief is a practice to do on your own—or maybe with a pet in the room—at home and not in a classroom situation. And before you start, a good idea is take the time to set up your environment to make it as comfortable as possible for you. Make sure you're practicing on a rug or mat, or even on a bed, and not a hard, cold floor. And set the lighting to whatever feels right for you.

In all poses, if it's cold, dress warmly and consider covering yourself with a blanket, It's also up to you whether you close your eyes in the poses or keep them open, partially or completely, with a soft gaze.

Because you need to be as comfortable as possible for more than just a few minutes, good choices for this practice are supported, symmetrical positions, including restorative poses and comfortable versions of Savasana.

If you already have an "old friend" pose that you feel comfortable in and/or comforted by, by all means choose that one. If you're not sure what to choose, it may be that the prone restorative poses—where you are facing down toward the floor rather than up toward the ceiling—will be the most comforting because people tend to feel safest in these poses. Here are some suggestions:

Supported Child's pose

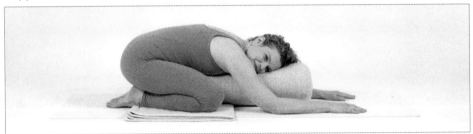

Prone Savasana

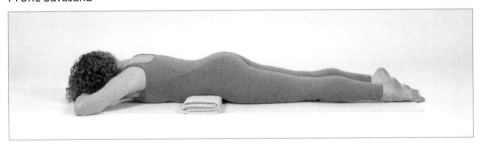

Supported Seated Forward Bend with any leg position

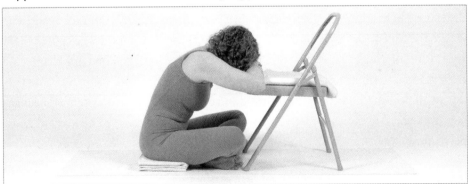

Desk Forward Bend

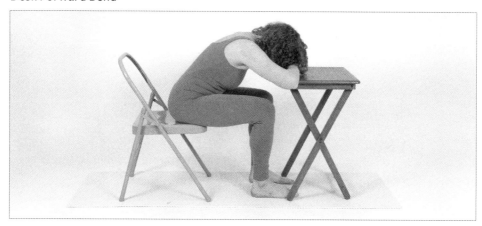

But another option is supported supine poses (in which you lie on your back) where your head and chest are lifted on a support. The support will open your chest a bit, inviting in a deeper breath, which could help let in some "light." But for some who are grieving—or who are in certain phases of grieving—even a gentle backbend like this can feel like too much. So use them at your discretion. Covering yourself with a blanket in these poses may make you feel less vulnerable.

Reclined Crossed-Legs pose

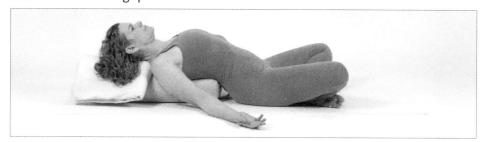

Reclined Cobbler's pose

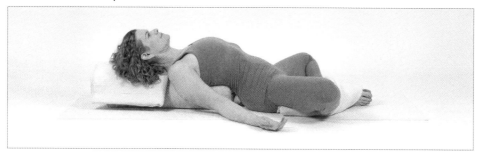

Supported Savasana

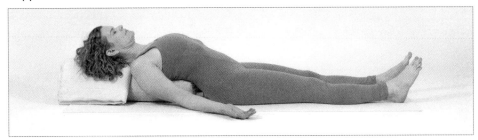

If you want to create a mini sequence of these poses, you can combine them anyway you wish or add in other comforting poses. Here's a suggestion:

Supported Child's pose

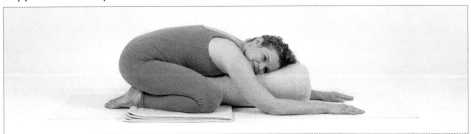

Supported Prone Twist (for equal amounts of time on each side)

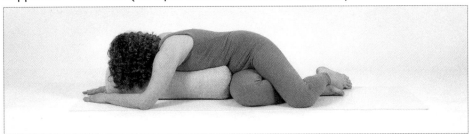

Supported Savasana of any kind

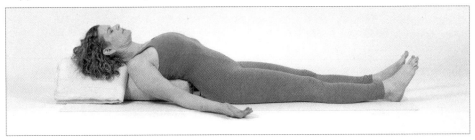

For those who have a regular seated meditation practice, or if you simply prefer to sit instead of doing a yoga pose, you can use a comfortable yoga seated position as you would for meditation or even sit on a chair.

WITNESSING GRIEF WITH MINDFULNESS

In the pause of just recognizing what you are feeling, you immediately transform from being overtaken by an emotion to experiencing a moment. In that pause, you recognize the temporary nature of your grief. In that pause, you see the light in your dark situation and see that time will help.

—Erin Collins, "A Hospice Nurse on Yoga for Grief," *Yoga for Healthy Aging Blog*

The practice of witnessing your grief or "holding space" for grief consists of nonjudgmentally observing your thoughts, emotions, and physical sensations, rather than trying to push them away. Basically, this practice is a form of mindfulness meditation. (Maybe the reason people these days call this practice "holding space" is to make the practice seem more approachable?)

Jivana Heyman says that after his mother died, when he returned to his meditation practice, his practice became an "exploration of feelings" more than a focused or directed practice: "I seek out that neutral field somewhere in my heart and rest there as I explore my feelings and thoughts, offering myself a loving presence and learning to mother myself."[7]

If you're already a practitioner of this type of meditation, witnessing your grief will be similar to the practice of witnessing any intense emotion. But if you're not familiar with mindfulness meditation and want to learn more, see How to Practice Mindfulness Meditation in chapter 7.

For grief, a mindfulness practice allows you *to fully feel* your grief in a safe and comfortable way, which can help you move through it. Robin Sturis, who is a clinical mental health counselor and yoga teacher, says that she practiced "holding space" this way for her own grief. And because she found it so helpful, she now offers the same assistance to others. She says that with regular practice, the difficult feelings become easier to hold. "With time they pass through us more smoothly, can even become friends—or at least familiar and less overwhelming visitors."[8]

And because one of the aims of mindfulness meditation is to learn to see reality as it is—impermanent and ever changing—and to make peace with this reality, the practice may help you accept your grief. Bonnie says that after the death of her youngest child, in the end she realized, "My grief will be a part of who I am for the rest of my life. It is how I continue to hold my son close."[9]

Mindfulness meditation is also intended to allow you to observe how your mind works, so the practice may help you identify good ways to support yourself. Notice if you are feeling anxious or scared, stressed or depressed, or even angry. Notice if you are physically agitated and restless or tired and lethargic. Simply acknowledge what you are feeling and accept that, without judgment. Later, if you wish, you can address these specific conditions with an asana practice such as those described in chapter 4.

Although I describe how to practice mindfulness meditation in general in chapter 7, a good way to practice for grief might be:

1. Start by practicing a few minutes of breath awareness to settle in.
2. When you're ready, allow yourself to focus on the grief you're experiencing. Notice whatever emotions, thoughts, and physical sensations arise. For each emotion, thought, or sensation that you observe, simply acknowledge it and accept it. This alone may reduce the intensity.
3. Turn your awareness to your body. Where is your grief centered in your body? What physical sensations are arising? Yoga and mindfulness meditation teacher Charlotte Bell says that turning your focus to the sensations in your body can allow you to disconnect from the "story" of your grief as you continue to feel it.
4. If a feeling is particularly intense, you could try intentionally reducing its intensity by using your breath. On your inhalation, bring awareness to your emotion. Then, on your exhalation, release that feeling out with your breath.
5. Feel free to stop any time you wish. You can return to breath awareness temporarily and then resume your grief practice, or you can end the practice with a few minutes of breath awareness or even just a few breaths.

You can also use this technique to "hold space" for others who are grieving. As they move through their grief, do your best to be fully present for them—without judgment, without trying to fix anything, and without any expectations for an outcome. Robin Sturis says:

Many people have never had this experience. It can be moving and transformative. It helps us to begin to see that we have value in our own right, that we are worthy of love and acceptance and that we can choose to be with ourselves in a way that is likely different than anything we have previously experienced.[10]

WITNESS GRIEF WITH A CONCENTRATION MEDITATION

I know my mother's love is still with me even though she is gone, but sometimes I forget and feel lost. So now I'm trying to find ways to unearth that love for myself, which can be surprisingly hard.

It's only through practice that I can remind myself that it's safe to be love instead of constantly trying to get love.

—Jivana Heyman, "The Life of Death: Finding the Eternal in the Temporary,"
Accessible Yoga Blog

After Jivana Heyman's mother died, besides practicing mindfulness in his exploration of his feeling as I described earlier, he also used the simple mantra "I love you" to connect to his mother's love. Inspired by this story, when I couldn't express my feelings in person to someone important to me who was dying, I used a simple mantra "I wish you peace" for him in my daily meditation practice.

This is a traditional yoga concentration practice, in which you use a mantra either to quiet your mind or to intentionally cultivate a particular state of mind, such as compassion, love, or gratitude. I provide detailed information about mantra meditation under How to Practice Concentration Meditation in chapter 7. But I wanted to mention the practice here because I myself found it so helpful for grief.

If you would like to use a mantra in this way, you can use any wording that you like or any mantra that you know. There are so many possibilities. You could express gratitude to someone for what they've given you or you could do a loving-kindness meditation for others who are suffering. On the other hand, if you need to forgive someone, you can practice the yama kshama, or if you need to let go of painful feelings, such as anger, that aren't serving you, you can practice letting go. (For information on forgiveness and letting go, see Letting Go on page 234.)

1. Start by practicing a few minutes of breath awareness to settle in.
2. When you are ready, picture the person or people you feel grief for in your mind's eye, and in your mind slowly say your chosen phrase.
3. Repeat the phrase as you continue to picture the person or people. If you wish, you can combine the phrase with breath awareness, by repeating the phrase once with each exhalation.
4. When your mind wanders, just notice it—refraining from making judgments about how well you are concentrating—and then return to the image again and repeat the phrase.
5. Continue for as long as you like.
6. Then, if it's comfortable for you to do so, sit quietly and notice how you feel.

Supporting Your Body, Mind, and Heart

Also, there are some common physical manifestations of grief such as fatigue, a sense of heaviness, anxiety, and lack of motivation, which I believe the practice of yoga can support and even improve. I believe each of our emotions has an energy that presides in the body. Yoga, with its movement and focus on the mind-body connection, can support an individual's experience of their personal grief response.

—Bonnie Maeda, "Grief and Yoga: An Interview with Bonnie Maeda, RN,"
Yoga for Healthy Aging Blog

Grief is not only a set of different "feelings," it also affects your body and your mind. It's especially common to feel fatigue, a sense of heaviness, and lack of motivation. It's also common to feel anxiety and experience a racing mind and to have physical symptoms related to anxiety, such as insomnia, poor digestion, and others. People may also feel anger, depression, or stress, along with related physical symptoms for those conditions.

Fortunately, you can use any of the yoga techniques I described in chapters 2 through 4 when you are experiencing grief. For example, in chapter 4, I mentioned that Jivana Heyman described feeling anxious after his mother's death, so he avoided quieter practices initially and practiced active yoga poses to address his anxiety. And Beth Gibbs told me that because she needed rest after her husband died, so although she continued to do her regular, active asana practice after her husband died, she spent more time than she previously had practicing Savasana and yoga nidra.

To support your body, mind, and heart, look for those practices that can help you address what you're currently experiencing but that also feel like something you can manage at that moment. Stress management of some kind might be particularly beneficial because reducing stress levels can help with many of the physical symptoms associated with grief, such as insomnia and poor digestion. And reducing your stress levels may reduce the intensity of some of your emotions. As always, though, everyone is different, so you should go with whatever appeals to you. And if something you try isn't working for you, just try something else.

Because fatigue and lethargy are so common for people who are grieving, I decided to offer an additional sequence in this section to complement the others in this book. This sequence is designed to energize you just a bit without overstimulating you. You can practice it on its own or use it as a prelude to any active practice that is in this book or elsewhere.

I also want to mention that Bonnie says that breath awareness can be an important aspect of moving through grief because bringing attention to your breath "encourages the life force of prana to be felt."[11] Erin Collins even says that she often advises students and families of the dying that taking three long, slow breaths "can turn a moment of deep sadness into a moment of transition."[12] You can practice breath awareness on its own or while you practice your yoga poses. If focusing on your breath makes you anxious, however, it's best to avoid that practice until you feel ready for it. See Coping Skill 1: Centering Yourself with Breath Awareness on page 17 for information on how to practice breath awareness.

Fatigue Practice

In this sequence, use your breath as a mental focus, if possible. Cover yourself with a blanket in pose 1. If you feel up to doing some active poses after practicing this, you could practice Moving Through Grief Practice on page 162 or Taking a Break from Grief Practice on page 166. Or you could just go about your day.

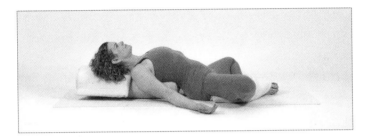

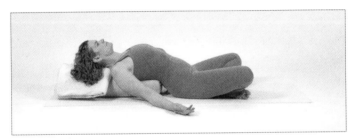

1. Supported Reclined Cobbler's pose or Reclined Crossed-Legs pose, *5 to 20 minutes*

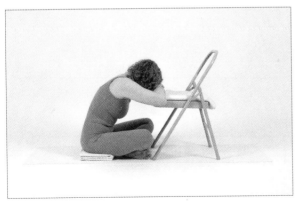

2. Supported Easy Sitting Forward Bend, *3 to 5 minutes*

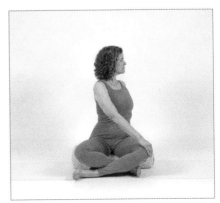

3. Easy Seated Twist,
   30 to 60 seconds per side

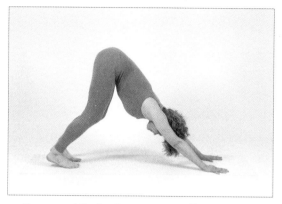
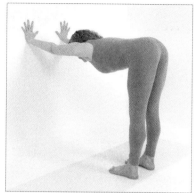

4. Downward-Facing Dog pose or Half Downward-
   Facing Dog pose, *30 to 60 seconds*

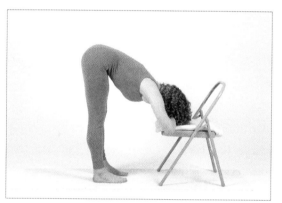
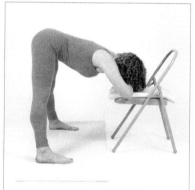

5. Supported Standing Forward Bend or Supported
   Wide-Legged Standing Forward Bend, *1 to 3 minutes*

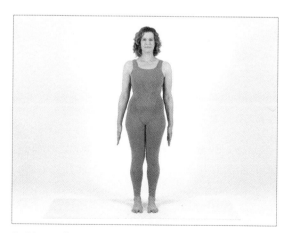

6. Mountain pose, *30 to 60 seconds*

Moving Through Grief

A full yoga experience of whatever style wakes you up to your feelings and attaches you to your body/mind is key.
—Dr. Lynn Somerstein, "Grief and Yoga: An Interview with
Dr. Lynn Somerstein," *Yoga for Healthy Aging Blog*

Although you might not feel up to practicing the way you used to do, when you're ready, using your asana practice to keep moving physically can be very helpful when you're grieving. An active asana practice, even a gentle one, can create a feeling of vitality. Beth Gibbs says continuing with her active practice after her husband's death helped release tension from her body, balanced her breath and energy, and calmed her mind so she could view what was happening clearly and "less through a victim, 'why me, why now' lens."

An active practice may be especially helpful if you're feeling stuck, something that Bonnie Maeda experienced after her son's death. She says, "I actually remember the day I said to myself, 'I don't want to live with this pain for the rest of my life.' At the same time, I did not know how not to. I was stuck."[13]

Now she believes that grief can be held in the body and that by practicing yoga poses there can be a "softening" or "spaciousness" in the areas where you're holding grief, so she teaches gentle stretching and supported vinyasas in her Yoga for Grief classes.

In general, releasing physical tension as described under Coping Skill 6: Releasing Physical Tension by Stretching in chapter 2 can make you feel calmer as well as more physically comfortable. Dr. Somerstein says that for grief, stretching your hip joints in particular releases "stored bound energy." You can stretch your hip joints by using any standing poses, seated poses, or reclined stretches where you take one or two legs out to the side, one leg behind you and one leg in front of you, and/or one leg across the midline of your body.

However, you may want to modify your practice during this time, especially if you're low on energy. Here are some suggestions:

1. **Choose easy poses or easy versions of poses.** Although the specific poses differ from person to person, almost everyone has poses they find easier to do and others that are more challenging. Now is the time to indulge yourself and focus on the ones that you like best. If you're practicing a sequence from this book, feel free to skip over a pose you just don't want to do.

2. **Use extra support.** If your energy is low, consider using extra support in active poses. For example, you could practice standing poses with your heel against the wall as shown throughout this book or you could use a chair to support your hands, for example, using your bottom hand in Triangle pose or both hands in Downward-Facing Dog pose. See chapter 6 for ideas about ways to modify your poses.

3. **Use shorter timings.** Before you start practicing, choose a shorter time than usual for holding active poses. But also monitor your energy levels as you start to practice. If you feel too tired to stay in a pose, just come out! If it's the first side of an asymmetrical pose, you can rest as described in number 5. Then do the second side for the same amount of time as you held the first side.

4. **Move with your breath.** Vinyasas, where you move between poses with your breath, can be particularly helpful during times of grief. They help keep your mind anchored in your body and can be energizing and even uplifting. Just be sure to move slowly between poses and take extra breaths in the poses themselves as needed. See Moving Through Grief Practice on page 162 for a suggested sequence.

5. **Rest as needed.** If at any time you feel like you just need to rest, there are some good poses you can use for resting during your practice. My suggestions are:

   - Mountain pose between standing poses
   - Easy Sitting pose between seated poses
   - Savasana between reclined poses
   - Child's pose (Balasana) between any poses

If you need to stop practicing entirely, it's a good idea to finish up with a symmetrical pose, whether Standing Forward Bend, Savasana, or Legs Up the Wall pose.

You may also want to use a phased approach to return to your asana practice. For example, Bonnie says that in the initial stage of grief, you could just lie on your mat and practice some stretches and perhaps try Supported Child's pose. Later on in the process, you could add in a few standing poses with short holds and maybe experiment with gentler backbends, such as a low Supported Bridge pose. Allow yourself to progress slowly and mindfully, depending on the amount of energy you have and your ability to focus. And keep in mind that the grief process is not linear, so there may be days when you need to do less than you did the day before. As part of each practice ask yourself, "How am I feeling in this moment, and what does my body need?"

Moving Through Grief Practice

This sequence is a gentle version of a mini Sun Salutation, in which you use a chair for your hands instead of the floor. This provides all the benefits of moving with your breath while reducing the energy needed to perform the classic version. In the first round, for step 4 step your left foot back into Lunge pose, and for step 6 step your left foot forward. After completing the sequence on your right side, return to step 1 and repeat on the left side by stepping back with your right foot in step 4 and forward with your right foot in step 6.

If the mini version is too short, after step 5, add Plank pose (Phalankasana), Upward-Facing Dog pose (Urdhva Mukha Svanasana), and a second Downward-Facing Dog pose, all with your hands on the chair, and then resume at step 6.

If you're exhausted before you practice, you could start with the Fatigue Practice on page 158. And if you want to move more slowly, move between the poses with your breath but stay in the poses themselves longer, for a few breaths instead of just one.

If you want to do more rounds, repeat steps 1 through 9 on both your right and left sides any number of times.

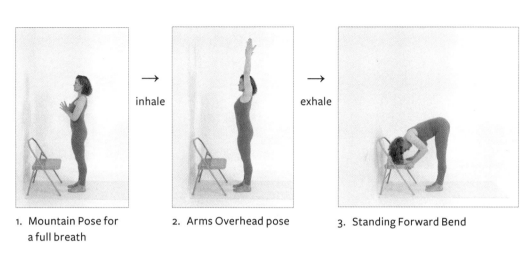

1. Mountain Pose for   2. Arms Overhead pose   3. Standing Forward Bend
   a full breath

 inhale

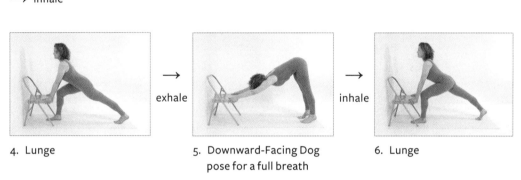

4. Lunge   5. Downward-Facing Dog   6. Lunge
                               pose for a full breath

→ exhale

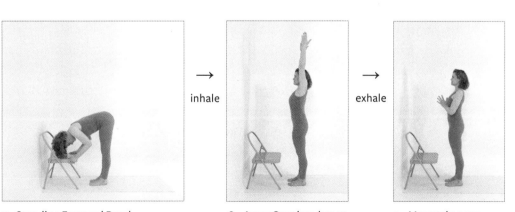

7. Standing Forward Bend   8. Arms Overhead pose   9. Mountain pose

Taking a Break from Grief

During periods of grief there may be days when you are craving a time out. This could be a protective mechanism because your pain feels overwhelming or because you're just tired out. A yoga practice that engages your mind as well as your body may be able to provide you with a safe way to take this type of temporary time-out.

If you're very fatigued or don't feel like doing an active practice, a guided relaxation practice such as yoga nidra, where a teacher's voice provides instructions that involve both your body and mind, can reduce your stress levels at the same time it is keeping your mind anchored in the here and now.

But if you want to do an active practice, as I described in Coping Skill 5: Taking a Break with a Mindful Asana Practice in chapter 2, there are many ways you can practice asanas with a mental focus, including using any of your five senses as well as proprioception and interoception. These will engage your mind as well as your body, which makes your asana practice a moving meditation.

For this type of practice, you could choose old-friend poses or an old-friend sequence that is easy to practice and that you know tends to make you feel better. Or you might want to try something new, as long as it's not something that scares you or makes you feel unsafe. Then, use any of the options for a mental focus that I describe under How to Practice Poses Mindfully in chapter 2. A good idea might be try something new to you because it will take more concentration—unless that is too frustrating.

In this context, practicing with a mental focus is a concentration practice rather than a mindfulness practice, because the aim is *not* to explore where your mind wanders off to. Instead, when you notice your mind has wandered, without judgment, simply return it to your mental focus. And as always practice nonjudgment, as well as self-compassion, with regard to how well you think you are concentrating. Finally, if you need to stop practicing entirely, do that without judgment too. It's a good idea, though, for your body's sake, to finish up with a symmetrical pose, whether Standing Forward Bend, Savasana, or Legs Up the Wall pose, if you can.

I decided to create an example sequence that you can try for this type of practice. This particular sequence is designed to open your chest, inviting in a deeper breath, which can be beneficial for those who are grieving. To practice this sequence for a brief respite, I'm suggesting that you use your proprioception—the sixth sense that allows you to feel how your body is moving in space—by moving and sensing your collarbones and shoulder blades in all the poses.

An alternative that might help you to "get out of yourself" is to practice using your sense of sight by gazing at something in nature, such as a tree, rock, or flower. You can do this when practicing outside or even by looking out of a window.

Taking a Break from Grief Practice

In this sequence, you'll move your awareness away from what you're thinking and feeling to your upper chest, both front and back. In every pose, focus on moving your collarbones away from each other and firming your shoulder blades against your back. Does this open your chest? Is it easier to maintain good posture? Are you able to take a deeper breath? When your mind wanders away from your collarbones and shoulder blades, simply return without judgment to the focus for this practice.

If you're fatigued before you practice, you could start with the Fatigue Practice on page 158.

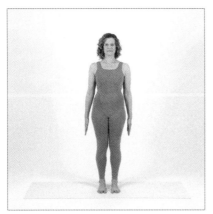

1. Mountain pose, *30 to 60 seconds*

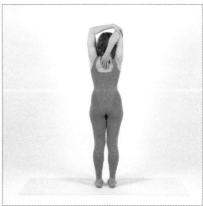

2. Standing Half-Cow Face pose, *30 to 60 seconds per side*

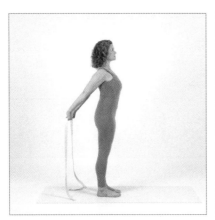

3. Standing Locust pose, *30 to 60 seconds per side*

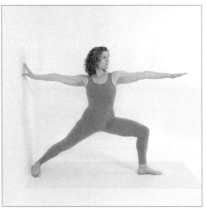

4. Warrior 2 pose, *30 to 60 seconds per side*

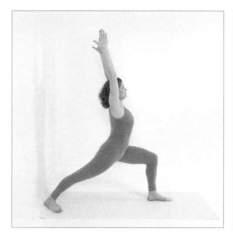

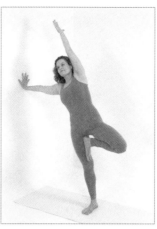

5. Warrior 1 pose,
   30 to 60 seconds per side

6. Wall Side Plank pose,
   30 to 60 seconds per side

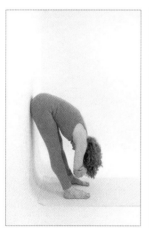

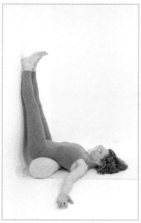

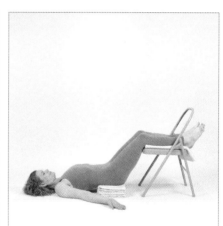

7. Wall Standing Forward
   Bend, *1 to 3 minutes*

8. Legs Up the Wall pose or Easy Inverted pose, *5 to 20 minutes*

6

Adapting to Physical Changes

Creating variations on poses and personalizing asana practice is about honoring the unique human bodies we are bringing to the mat. Bodies change from day to day (minute to minute, even!) and throughout the seasons of our lives. Honoring the body you bring to the mat today by treating your body with kindness, compassion, and ally-ship (as opposed to something to be subjugated or "fixed") is a way of practicing ahimsa (nonviolence) and satya (truthfulness) together. Personalizing your practice is powerful!

—Amber Karnes, yoga teacher and founder of
Body Positive Yoga, *Accessible Yoga Blog*

No matter what your current physical condition is, continuing to be physically active is so important for your mental and emotional health as well as your physical health. Fortunately, yoga is so adaptable—the full spectrum of practice includes so many possibilities between a full active practice of classic poses and chair yoga—that there will almost always be something you can do.

Tracey was thirty and in excellent health when she sprained her ankle while she was dancing. During the four months that it took her ankle to heal, she practiced her standing poses seated in a chair, both at home and in public classes. She said that it actually turned out to be a wonderful experience. She had a lot of fun figuring out different ways to practice using the chair, plus having a temporary (and minor) disability enabled her to experience more compassion for those who are facing all types of health challenges.

On the other hand, by late middle age, my friend Ariel began developing osteoarthritis in both knees and later in her hips. A longtime yoga practitioner, she kept practicing yoga poses by customizing her poses. In standing poses with bent knees, she no longer bent her knees to 90 degrees, but backed off quite a bit to avoid stressing her knee joints. In seated and reclined poses, she used props under her outer legs to support her hip joints and to keep the muscles around them from overstretching. Ultimately, to keep some of the weight off her joints, she began practicing standing poses with her back against a yoga horse or a wall and kept her feet closer together than in the classic versions. Now she says:

> I had to give up ballet, which I loved, because that had a limited lifespan for me. But now with yoga it is so reassuring that the poses can be adapted to allow me to continue to practice no matter what is going on.[1]

So, whether you need to *change* the way you're doing yoga poses or if you started doing yoga *because* of a physical change, the ability to customize poses will allow you to find ways to practice that work with your new reality. Rather than illustrating all the different ways of doing every pose you might want to do—which would actually be impossible—this chapter will suggest some basic techniques—such as changing the orientation of a yoga pose—that you can use to come up with variations of your own.

From my own experience with physical changes, both temporary (a frozen shoulder) and permanent (osteoarthritis), it has been so empowering to come up with my own customizations. These not only enabled me to keep my practice going when I could no longer do what I used to do, but I was reassured to know that when the future brings other physical changes I'll be able to adapt and adjust to them as well.

In this chapter, I'll provide many suggestions for how to adapt yoga poses to your current physical condition. You can use those adaptations for any of the poses in this book or any poses in any sequence that you want to practice.

Practicing with Wisdom

Before I share my suggestions for how to customize your yoga poses, here are some basic guidelines for choosing and practicing your poses when you have a physical limitation of some kind, whether temporary or permanent. I'll conclude with a short section about what you can do when—for any reason—you can't practice yoga poses at all.

FOCUS ON SAFETY

If you're customizing your practice because of an illness or physical problem and you don't already know the contraindications for your condition, start by doing some research. Ask your doctor or physical therapist about movements that are okay for you and those that are not. Don't just ask whether "yoga" is okay, but go through the list of the various movements you plan to make, such as forward bending, back bending, twisting, arms overhead, partial and full inversions, and so on. Then, when you practice, you'll know which types of movements and positions you should not be doing. See the appendix, Tips for Staying Safe, for more information.

TAKE A YOGIC APPROACH

To adapt your asana practice to physical changes in a yogic way I suggest you practice both *arjava* (honesty) and skill in action. Taking this kind of yogic approach will not only help you find the poses that are best for your current condition, but it will also help you stay calm and steady through the process.

Arjava. One of the ten yamas mentioned in the Yoga Yajnavalkya, Hatha Yoga Pradipika, and other yoga texts, arjava (honesty) is the practice of being truthful with yourself and respecting what is actually happening for you at this moment in time. So, as you decide how to adapt your practice and then start practicing the poses you've chosen, observe how you think and how you feel without shame or any kind of judgment. This can help you realize when you're taking on more than you can handle or when fears are holding you back. (See Practicing Self-Inquiry on page 236 for more information on arjava.)

Skill in action. Practicing skill in action means focusing solely on the action you're taking, without worrying about what the end results will be. It also means accepting the results of your action, whether success or failure, with equanimity. This is the yogic approach to all actions that is the message at the heart of the Bhagavad Gita. So when you try out a new variation of a pose, try approaching it with a sense of curiosity. And if you realize the variation isn't working for you, see if you can simply let it go and try something else instead. (See Taking Action on page 254 for more information on skill in action.)

PRACTICE WITH MINDFULNESS

Practicing mindfully can help you stay safe as you find the best pose for you at this time. Practicing yoga poses with mindfulness means nonjudgmentally observing what happens in your body as you practice. When you experiment with a new yoga pose or a new version of a yoga pose, practicing mindfulness can help you determine whether or not the pose is right for you. It can be particularly helpful to pay attention to your breath. Is your breathing ragged or labored? Or is it relatively easy and natural? And it can also be helpful to tune in to any pain you feel, especially around your joints. Difficulty breathing and pain around your joints can be warning signals that you either need to ease off or stop what you're doing and choose another variation or another pose instead.

BE OPEN TO PROPS AS WELL AS VARIATIONS

Some yoga practitioners don't want to use props because they've been told it is "cheating." But the truth is that yoga props are traditional in India and were always considered beneficial. Early statues of yoga practitioners show them with straps around their legs to steady them in seated poses. And in *The Yoga Sutras of Patanjali*, Edwin Bryant says that one of the poses from more than 1,500 years ago was Soprasaya, the Support pose. Although there are differing opinions about what sort of prop was used, Bryant says that this support pose indicates that "props have been used for centuries and are, in this sense, authentic."[2]

Props are so useful for adapting poses to your particular body type as well as to your current physical condition; I hope that you'll open your mind to them if you aren't already using them.

WHEN YOU CAN'T PRACTICE

Yoga is also accessible on my worst days. Observing my body, mind and spirit without judgment can be challenging. When I allow myself that experience, though, I know I tend to feel better.

—Cherie Hotchkiss, "Bed-Bound Yoga," *Accessible Yoga Blog*

If there is ever a time when it's not possible for you to practice any yoga poses, even customized ones, there are still two things you can do to have an embodied yoga experience, even if you are limited to practicing in bed.

1. **Savasana.** You can stay connected to your body by practicing any form of Savasana with a body scan, where you focus on progressively relaxing the different parts of your body, one by one, or you can practice any form of breath awareness. Cherie Hotchkiss, a yoga teacher who has been managing a diagnosis of multiple sclerosis for over twenty years, says that Savasana is her go-to practice when she is "bed bound."

2. **Imagining your practice.** If you miss your asana practice, you can try practicing it mentally. My friend Carol, a longtime yoga practitioner, told me that after sustaining a severe neck injury she spent a couple of months where her movements were very restricted. Because she had read that just imagining making specific movements with your body could help you retain muscle memory, she did her daily yoga practice in bed by imagining that she was practicing each of the poses in her sequence, one by one. She said that she felt this way of practicing did help her retain muscle memory, and also helped her maintain her image of herself as "healthy and strong."

Customizing Poses

There is a myth about yoga poses—which some modern teachers even promote—that the poses are ancient and perfect and that you should never do them differently from the way you were taught. But the truth is that most of what we do in modern yoga was developed by innovative Indian teachers in the early twentieth century, including Krishnamacharya and B. K. S. Iyengar. And this is one of the reasons why there is always more than one way—or even three ways—to do a yoga pose.

You see, even the classic versions of many of the yoga poses vary among the different yoga traditions. Triangle pose is an excellent example of this. In the Iyengar tradition the feet are very wide apart, and the top arm is straight up toward the ceiling. In the Integral Yoga tradition the feet are much closer together, and the top arm is alongside the ear, not straight up to the ceiling. And in the Viniyoga version the feet are closer together, but the arm position is the same as in the Iyengar version.

Then there are the "official" variations of the classic poses that you can learn in yoga classes or see in so many books and videos. These not only vary from tradition to tradition but also from teacher to teacher. Many contemporary yoga teachers continue to make up variations.

So there's definitely no "sacred" one single way to do a pose. I hope this makes you feel more comfortable with the idea of customizing your own poses. I believe that even if you're not a yoga teacher, if you have some experience practicing a pose in a classroom setting and you follow the guidelines I suggested earlier, you can benefit from customizing a pose to suit your current physical condition as well as your body type. You might even enjoy the process.

TECHNIQUES FOR CUSTOMIZING A YOGA POSE

The other night when I was cooking dinner, I had an *epiphanette* (my word for a tiny epiphany). As usual, even though I had a recipe in front of me, the actual way I was making it was different in several ways from the written instructions. Over time, I'd been tinkering with the recipe by changing the amounts of certain ingredients and even adding a new one (almost any pasta sauce is better with some red-pepper flakes, right?) until I was finally satisfied with it. That's when I suddenly realized that customizing a yoga pose was very similar to tinkering with a recipe; with just a few simple tweaks, you can make it your own. This section provides six different strategies for customizing a yoga pose. While I don't always use the cooking metaphor for all six strategies, if you keep the idea of tinkering with a recipe in mind, it might make you more comfortable with the process.

You can use the following tips for customizing the poses in any of the sequences in this book or in any other sequence you want to practice.

Do the Pose More Gently

Take the basic shape of the pose but don't go as "deeply" into it as photos of the classic pose typically show it or as "deeply" as you used to practice it. For example, my favorite variation that I came up with is the gentler, more accessible version of Warrior 3 pose.

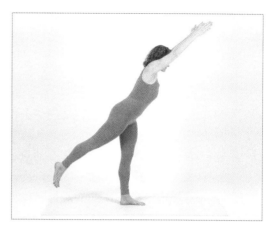

So in any pose, don't bend your hips, back, or knees as much. Don't stretch as far. Don't turn as far in a twist. Don't lift your leg as high. Don't take your legs as far apart. Don't bend as far in a forward bend—or keep your spine extended instead of rounding it. If you think of it as tinkering with a recipe, it's like reducing the salt, the oil, the hot pepper, or the garlic—all the ingredients are still there but maybe just not as much of some of them.

Using this technique sometimes can mean using a prop, for example, under your knees in a seated pose to keep your hips from overstretching or under your hands in a backbend so you don't bend as deeply. But other times it simply means backing off from the classic version. For example, many people with bad knees find it helpful to bend their knees less than 90 degrees in standing poses. My friend Ariel says that, in general, she has now stopped pushing herself and is becoming attuned to feeling good in the pose.

Change the Foundation of the Pose

The foundation of your pose is the part of your body that is touching the ground. Changing your foundation can make the pose steadier, gentler, or, in some cases, make more space for your body if there is a part that is feeling squished. If you think of this as tinkering with a recipe, maybe it's like replacing all that butter with some extra virgin olive oil—something I do all the time—to make the pose healthier for you.

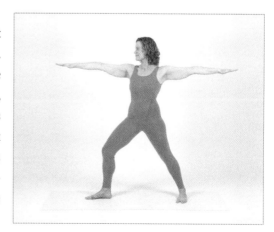

For standing poses—or any poses where your feet are on the ground—you can change the alignment of your feet. In a pose where the classic version has toes touching or feet very close together, try moving your feet apart, either in line with your hip joints or even further. This is how my friend Ariel practices to reduce the stress on her hip joints.

If you have a single foot near a different body part, such as in the seated twists Marichi's pose 3 (Marichyasana 3) and Half Lord of the Fishes pose (Ardha Matseyendrasana), try moving your foot further away. In a pose where the classic version has the feet very wide apart, try moving your feet closer together. In a pose where the classic version has the front foot aligned with the back foot in a heel-to-arch relationship, try widening out a bit, aligning heel to heel or even wider apart.

When you are kneeling and your shins are your foundation or part of it, try moving your shins a bit apart. When your hands or forearms are either the foundation or part of the foundation, you can also try moving them further apart to find more stability or room for your body.

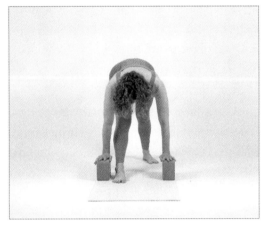

In some poses, your foundation is actually your hip points, as in Locust pose, or your sitting bones, as in Boat pose (Navasana). Of course, you can't move these bones further apart, but you can cushion them with a folded blanket, which can help make the pose gentler.

Remove an Element from the Pose

If there is a movement you cannot make, such as raising both arms or standing on two feet, you can do just do the part of the pose that's accessible to you. You can also remove an element from the classic pose to make the pose less physically demanding. If you think of it as tinkering with a recipe, it's like leaving out one of the ingredients entirely.

Although almost all standing poses involve both legs and arms, you can do them all keeping your arms at your sides or with your hands on your hips. For example, Warrior 1, 2, and 3 can all be done this way. On the other hand, you can also do arm positions without leg positions. For example, you can do arm positions for Eagle pose (Garudasana), Warrior 1 pose, and Warrior 2 pose while seated in a chair or with simple Mountain pose legs. To adapt Eagle pose for her knee condition, Ariel practices the arm position for Eagle pose with two feet on the floor and knees slightly bent.

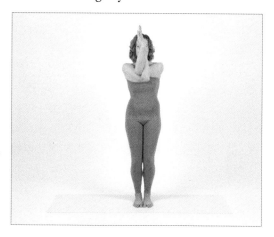

The same is true for seated poses that involve arm movements. For example, you can do just the legs or just the arms in Cow-Face pose. If you can't do the leg position in a seated pose, do the arm position with a leg position that does work for you. For seated forward bends that involve stretching your arms forward or down toward your feet, if you can't bring your arms alongside your ears, you can do just the leg and back positions as you find an alternate position for your hands that is comfortable for you.

Make Friends with a Wall

When you're practicing yoga at home, if you don't have a bare wall, make it a priority to clear one if at all possible. There are so many different ways to use it!

Back to the wall. Seated poses as well as standing poses can be practiced with your back or hips touching the wall for support and to make the pose gentler. Examples are Easy Sitting pose with your back against the wall, Standing Forward Bend with your buttocks

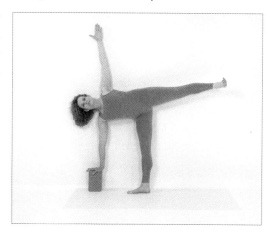

on the wall, and Half Moon pose (Ardha Chandrasana) with your hip and top hand on the wall. You can also practice standing poses near a wall for a feeling of security. For example, for those who have balance problems, practicing balance poses such as Tree pose (Vrksasana) and Eagle pose, or standing poses that have feet wide apart, such as Triangle pose and Extended Side-Angle pose (Utthita Parsvakonasana), with your back to a wall can be very reassuring.

Side to the wall. Seated twists, even done in a chair, as well as some standing poses can be practiced with your hands or another body part on the wall for support. Examples are Tree pose with your bent knee touching the wall and Noose pose (Pasasana) with hands on the wall.

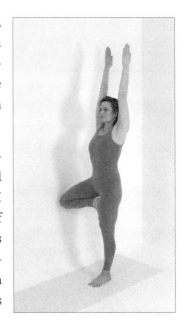

Front to the wall. Several standing poses, such as Pyramid pose, Warrior 1, and Warrior 3 can be practiced with your hands on the wall for support. Recently I practiced Camel pose (Ustrasana) with the fronts of my thighs on the wall, so I'm sure there are other poses you can do facing the wall. (See Changing the Orientation of a Pose later in this chapter for information about how you can use the wall as the "floor" for poses that are normally done on the floor.)

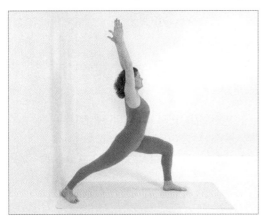

Heel or heels on the wall. A classic way to make wide-legged standing poses more stable and less demanding is to position your back heel against the wall with your front foot facing the middle of the room. This book shows many of the standing poses this way. For Downward-Facing Dog pose, you can practice with both heels up on the wall, which makes the pose steadier and less demanding.

Be Creative with Props

If the traditional props don't work for you because they're not the right shape or size, look around the house and see what you can find. You can use small household items, such as bath towels, hand towels, and washcloths, to provide just a bit of support, use books instead of blocks, use bags of rice or beans instead of sandbags, and so on. You can also use your furniture. I'll never forget hearing the yoga teacher

Patricia Walden say that every time she walked into a hotel room she did a quick inventory to see which furniture she could use in her practice. Ariel told me she found that the countertop in her kitchen was better than the wall for supporting herself in standing poses because she could place her hands on its surface. And one of the best uses of furniture I know of is using a dining table, sturdy coffee table, or firm bed as a "raised floor" for those who want to do reclined poses but can't get up and down from the floor.

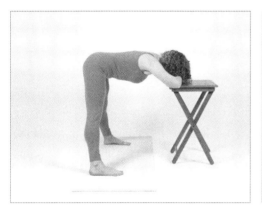 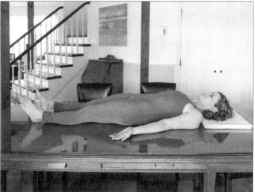

Change the Orientation of the Yoga Pose

For some people a whole category of poses is not accessible in their classic mode. Perhaps you can't stand up, can't get up and down from the floor, can stand up but can't lie down, can't bear weight on your hands, or can't go upside down. The solution to this is to change the orientation of the yoga pose. Once you get into the habit of seeing that the basic shape of a pose can be done standing, seated, reclined, or using the wall as the floor, you're sure to come up with a variation that suits you.

Although you won't get exactly the same physical benefits from the pose when you change its orientation, you will still be taking the basic shape of the pose, which can help you maintain flexibility and range of motion as well as strength. And taking a variety of shapes will help your coordination and fine-muscle control. It will also allow you to expand the repertoire of poses you can do so that you don't have to do just a few poses over and over.

The following section describes this technique in detail.

CHANGING THE ORIENTATION OF A POSE

One of my neighbors told me that her problem with yoga was that she couldn't do any poses lying down because she always felt nauseated when she was lying down. And when she consulted her doctor about it, her doctor told her just not to do them. I said to her, "You don't need to let that stop you! There are actually multiple ways you can do any yoga pose, so even if you can't lie down, you could do a given pose standing up instead, for example." I explained to her that an important basic principle regarding making a pose accessible was just to change the orientation of the pose! To my cooking metaphor, this is kind of like the time I took my children's favorite soup recipe, Risi e Bisi (rice and pea), and turned it into a rice and pea salad because it was summer. They liked it!

Yoga poses are classically divided into four groups: standing poses, seated poses, supine poses (on your back, same as the Sanskrit word *supta*), and prone poses (on your belly). It's helpful to think of these as different "modes" of practicing. For some, like my neighbor, all the poses in one of those modes aren't accessible. For example, maybe you can't stand up at all, so you can't do the classic versions of standing poses. Or maybe you can't get down to and up from the floor, so you can't do the classic versions of seated, supine, and prone poses. Or maybe you need to do all your poses seated in a chair.

When one of these modes of practicing isn't available to you, try changing its mode by practicing the basic shape of the pose in one of the modes that is accessible to you. In my neighbor's case, for example, she could do a pose we do lying down, Reclined Leg Stretch (Supta Padangusthasana), standing up instead by practicing Standing Leg Stretch (Utthita Hasta Padangusthasana) with the lifted leg supported by a chair or something higher, such as a countertop. For those in the opposite situation, you would do Reclined Leg Stretch lying down or seated in a chair instead of Standing Leg Stretch.

Sometimes, as in the case of Padangusthasana, a version of a given pose already exists in more than one orientation (if there are two poses with the same name but one begins with *supta* that gives you a clue). But when there isn't, you can just go ahead and make up a new variation. For example, for Cobra pose, which is normally done prone on the floor, someone (I wish I knew who!) created a really nice variation that you do standing with your hands on the wall.

When you start thinking along these lines, you'll find a way to do almost any pose. Using this technique will not only give you more poses to practice at home on your own but when you're in class it will allow you to figure out what to do on your own if your teacher is busy with something else and can't help you. When I had a frozen shoulder, I used this technique in class all the time.

Now let's take a closer look at four different ways you can change the orientation of a pose.

Lying Down

You can take the shape of many standing poses lying with your back on the floor with your feet on the wall, as if the wall were the floor and the floor were a wall. If you can't get up and down from the floor, you could use a yoga platform, a dining room table, a sturdy coffee table, or even a firm bed as your floor. For example, here is Arms Overhead pose on the floor.

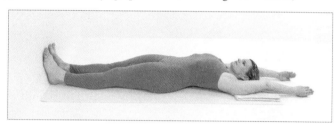

When you do the standing pose lying on the floor, rather than just resting against the floor in the shape of the pose, activate the same muscles that you would as if you were standing, so you're actively doing the pose. For example, in a reclined Tree pose, you would firm your "standing" foot into the wall as you press the foot of your bent leg toward your thigh and press your inner thigh toward the foot. Reach your arms overhead and activate them, as if you were reaching them up toward the ceiling.

For Handstand, you could practice by lying on the floor with your hands on a wall! Keep the image of the classic pose in your mind as you activate your entire body.

Seated on a Chair

You can generally take the shape of any standing or seated pose with either part or all of your body when you are seated on a chair. If you can move your legs, your legs can take the same shape they would if you were standing without putting weight on them. Although your pelvis is supported by the chair, you will still be working against gravity to hold yourself up, so a chair version of a standing pose can be surprisingly physically

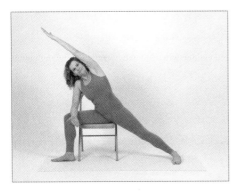

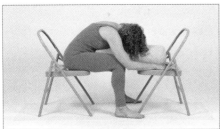

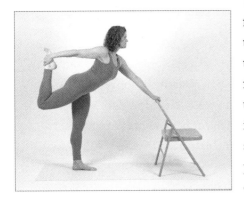

demanding (I have tried them!). See left for an example of Extended Side Angle pose.

For those who can't do supine or prone poses on the floor, you can often use two chairs and a lot of props to get into a close approximation of the pose. For example, shown here is a variation of Supported Child's pose practiced sitting in a chair.

Although some people who have a hard time getting up and down from the floor stop doing it entirely, I encourage you, if at all possible, to continue to practice some floor poses even if you need some help from a prop or wall in order to move down to the floor and up again. The same is true for people who need help of some kind to balance while standing up, whether that is from a cane or using hands on a chair. Even if it's very challenging for you, I think it's worth your effort to maintain the agility and balance you do have by continuing to work on both getting up and down from the floor and balancing on your feet rather than giving up entirely. So, if you regularly practice chair yoga, if at all possible, consider doing some floor and standing poses as well. The photo on the left shows practicing Dancer's pose (Natarajasana) with a chair to help with balance.

Standing

If you think of the wall as the floor, there are many prone poses, such as Cobra pose, that you can do standing with part of your body against the wall. For example, I can see doing Locust pose with your hip points against a wall and arms lifted behind you or Plank pose with either hands or forearms on the wall. In his book *Accessible Yoga*, Jivana Heyman has a wall version of the entire Sun Salutation that uses the wall as a floor!

One advantage of standing in front of the wall over lying on the floor is that there is less weight on your hands, so these variations are very good for those with problems in the wrists or hands. Half Downward-Facing Dog pose at the wall is the classic example of this, as is the wall version of Side Plank pose (Vasisthasana) with one hand on the wall, shown below.

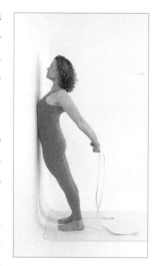

And because your orientation to gravity is different—you no longer have to lift yourself up away from the ground—these versions are less physically demanding, so they're good for those who have less energy or strength.

I can even imagine some supine poses against the wall, such as a passive backbend with a prop behind your shoulder blades and arms reaching up toward the ceiling or a wall version of Standing Leg Stretch (Hasta Padangusthasana) with your back against the wall to help with balancing.

Obviously relaxing reclined poses are not going to be relaxing if you do them standing up, so for restorative supine or most prone poses I would recommend using two chairs and a lot of props instead as mentioned earlier. Even better, you could use a yoga platform, a dining room table, a sturdy coffee table, or even a firm bed as your floor.

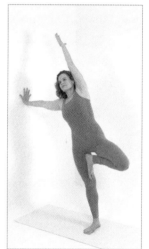

Upside Down versus Right Side Up

For those who cannot go upside down into a full inversion, if your condition allows it, you may be able to do a partial inversion in the form of a similar pose. For example, an alternative to Headstand is to do a Standing Forward Bend with your head on a block (or two) or with your head and arms on a chair or to do Wide-Legged Standing Forward Bend with head support. I did both of those when I had a frozen shoulder.

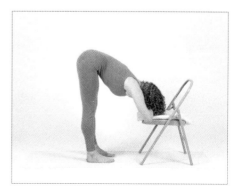

Instead of practicing Shoulderstand, you could do Supported Bridge pose—a much more gradual inversion that puts much less weight on your neck.

You can also try the pose right side up, such as Handstand with your feet on the floor and your hands in the air, as if they were touching the ceiling. I've seen fellow students doing that in class.

Customizing Your Practice

After you have customized your poses, you can use them in any of the sequences in this book or any other sequences that you want to practice. And if a pose in any sequence just isn't working for you at all, you can simply skip over it. Just practice the remaining poses in their original order.

But what if there are so many poses you can't do that this way of modifying sequences isn't satisfying to you? One of my readers once wrote to me with that problem. She had a foot injury and wanted an active practice that she could do without standing and without sitting in a chair. What she had been doing so far, she said, was just practicing poses "as they pop into my head." But she now realized that being more "systematic" about it might be a better way to go.

Rather that writing a sequence for her myself, which I easily could have done, I wanted to empower her to take care of herself. So I suggested that she do what I had done in a similar situation, with a different injury. She wrote me back saying she was very happy with my advice, so I'll suggest the same for you:

1. Do some research and make a list of all the poses you can do in your current condition.
2. Create two or more sequences from these poses—so you don't have to do the same thing every day—in the style of yoga that you typically do. These can either be balanced sequences containing a mixture of pose types, or they can be more focused practices such as a backbend practice, a forward-bend practice, or a twist practice.

Sequencing poses is an art, and the approach to it varies among the different yoga traditions. So I'm not going to try to go into details here about how to do it. But basically, most active sequences have three parts:

Warm-up poses. These poses are typically gentle stretches that prepare you for practicing the active poses, either by providing all-over stretching or by stretching the areas you're going to focus on in your active poses.

Active poses. These poses can be a mixture of different types of poses or they can focus on a single category of active poses, such as backbends, forward bends, twists, or inverted poses. Even when practicing a single type of pose, it's typical to start with easier active poses and gradually move to more challenging ones.

Cool-down poses. These poses allow you to release muscle tension created by the active practice. In some traditions, these are "counter-poses" to the active poses you practice. For example, after backbends or forward bends, you might practice a twist as a counter-pose. Typically the final "cool-down pose" is Savasana, which allows you to relax your body in anatomical neutral and calm down from any stimulation created by the practice. But if you don't like Savasana, you can choose any other symmetrical relaxing pose.

If you want more information about how to sequence poses, I suggest that you find some books or articles about sequencing in the tradition that you practice or see if your teacher has some ideas for you.

7

Being Present

Freedom means actually experiencing the divinity in each moment, which is
the same as not wanting the present moment to be any different from the
way it is. When you don't want any moment to be different, when you give
your heart's consent to what is, then you are no longer struggling (or even
waiting) for a better situation, and therefore you are free to fully show up for
what is actually happening now.
                    —Christopher D. Wallis, *Tantra Illuminated*

In chapter 1 I discussed how even though we evolved to plan for the future, there are
many times when this urge to plan isn't helpful and prevents us from facing the reality
of actually what's going on in the present. In *Tantra Illuminated* Christopher Wallis describes the four forms of grasping that he says prevent us from "immersing ourselves"
in the present moment:

> In the past we grasp toward positive memories, which is called nostalgic rev-
> erie, and we grasp after painful memories in the form of guilt and regret. We
> grasp future imaginary possibilities, which is called fantasy, and future nega-
> tive possibilities, which is called worry or anxiety.[1]

On the other hand, if you're anchored in the present, when something changes you won't be comparing the present with the past and feeling the loss or blaming yourself or others for how things turned out. And you won't be fantasizing or wishing that the future will bring the solutions to all your problems or miraculously set things back to the way they were in the past. Wallis says that when we let go of the four forms of grasping, "we let past and future become part of our present and experience the fullness of the present, which has much more to offer us that the mind could ever imagine."[2]

During the extreme fire season in California, I found it more challenging than ever to stay present. My mind raced into the future: Was there going to be a serious fire season every year from now on? Would we be able to continue living in California, where I previously thought we'd spend the rest of our lives? I caught myself worrying about the future pretty quickly and reminded myself of my "Don't panic too soon" motto. I came up with that motto back in the 1990s when I was working in the high-pressure environment of a small software startup company—the company would fail if we didn't get our product out on time—and I was in charge of the complete set of documentation! And that motto has helped me ever since. I also used my yoga practice during the extreme fire season to stay calm and be present with what was happening rather than panicking too soon. (Yes, "Don't panic too soon" is a play on the cover of *The Hitchhiker's Guide to the Galaxy*.)

My friend Melitta Rorty says something similar. When she notices that she is stressed about the future or ruminating about the past, she brings/drags herself into the present just by saying to herself, "This present moment is perfect, there is nothing wrong here," and in less than a minute, this leads her to a calmer state. But I think that the little phrases Melitta and I use to remind ourselves to be present only work because she and I have been practicing yoga for decades. Through our practices, we have learned to bring ourselves back to the present, over and over, when we notice that our minds are drifting off into the future or the past.

That's why I'm dedicating a chapter to pranayama and meditation: both are powerful practices for training you to be present because of the concentration they require. Practicing either one—or both—can help you become more present in your everyday life because you will develop the habit of noticing when your mind is wandering. And the more you practice returning your focus to the present, the stronger your habit will become, both in the yoga room and in your life.

In this chapter, I'll start by discussing pranayama first because in traditional yoga pranayama is seen as the gateway to meditation. However, you don't necessarily have to practice pranayama before you meditate. If you're not yet practicing either one, read through both sections and see what appeals to you the most at this time.

Breath Practices (Pranayama)

Pranayama is the traditional yogic practice of conscious breathing. Rather than just letting your breath come naturally, with pranayama you use various techniques to slow your breath, pause your breath, speed up your breath, breathe through alternate nostrils, and so on. Because we normally breathe without thinking about it, intentionally changing the way you breathe, especially for an extended period of time, takes a lot of concentration! So breath practices are a good way to yoke your body and mind to the present moment. Focusing on your internal sensations will settle your mind, and being present will take your mind off regrets about the past and worries about the future.

But pranayama can be more powerful than you might think, and there two are very different ways to use it in your daily life:

1. **As a concentration practice.** Pranayama hones your ability to focus in general and provides a gateway to meditation.
2. **As a self-regulation practice.** Pranayama provides you with a key to your nervous system that you can use to directly affect your moods and energy levels.

Understanding these two different ways of using pranayama is important, because this will help you to select the breath practices that are right for you and to avoid the practices that aren't.

A GATEWAY TO MEDITATION

Pranayama is not only an instrument to steady the mind, but also the gateway to concentration, *dharana*.

—B. K. S. Iyengar, *Light on the Yoga Sutras of Patanjali*

Pranayama (breath practices), along with meditation, was one of the earliest yoga practices in ancient India. In that era, it was used to purify the mind and body, build self-discipline, and settle the mind before meditation. According to Georg Feuerstein, the Shvetashvatara-Upanishad instructed that "conscious breathing should begin as a prelude to meditation."[3] In modern times, we are taught that pranayama is one of the branches in the eightfold path in Classical Yoga (the yoga of Patanjali's Yoga Sutras) as well as in other yoga paths, and that pranayama always precedes the first stage of meditation to prepare your mind and body for yoga's higher practices. Breath practices also hone your ability to focus, a skill needed for meditation and many other yoga practices as well as for staying present in your everyday life.

You can use pranayama as a prelude to a meditation session to settle your mind before you start meditating. I have more than one friend who begins every meditation session by practicing Alternate Nostril Breath, a form of pranayama that requires quite a bit of concentration. You can also include pranayama as part of a sequence of yoga poses. For example, you might begin an asana session with a brief session of pranayama to help settle you in the present moment or end with your asana practice with a session of pranayama to prepare you for your final Savasana. And of course you can do pranayama on its own at any time of the day.

For those who are not ready for meditation or who just do not want to meditate for any reason, practicing pranayama might be a good alternative because a structured breath practice is especially engaging for your mind. The same is true if you are depressed or anxious and you find that meditation causes you to spiral down into a troubling place.

However, because some people find focusing on their breathing makes them anxious, as with any yoga practice, if you find that breath practices are not working for you for any reason, you should skip them. Instead, try meditating with a mantra or consider a guided meditation where you can follow the instructions given by a teacher (see How to Practice Concentration Meditation on page 208).

Because breath practices can have a strong effect on your nervous system, when choosing a breath practice to settle your mind before meditating or as a way to sharpen your focus, you may want to use practices such as Equal Ratio Breath (Sama Vrtti) and Alternate Nostril Breath (Nadi Shodana) that have inhalations and exhalations of the same length. Those practices will have the mildest effect on your moods and energy levels. However, if you want to slightly stimulate yourself when you're feeling drowsy or calm yourself when you're feeling hyper, see Breath Practices for Self-Regulation on page 191 for suggested breath practices that you can use to balance yourself.

In a Tantra Yoga tradition, you can use the pause at the end of your breath cycles to experience the single divine consciousness of which we are all a part. First, choose a breath practice where you intentionally lengthen the pause at the end of your exhalation (the *bahya kumbhaka*) by a comfortable amount (see Calming Breath Practice: Extending the Exhalation on page 197). Then, within each pause, rest there in the present, experiencing the quietness that underlies all the activity and change inherent in everyday life or just experience a moment of deep peace. In her book *Meditation for the Love of It*, Sally Kempton describes it this way:

> Letting yourself stay in that moment of emptiness at the end of the exhalation is a way of entering into the space of the Self. Notice how in that space you are fully in the present. There is no past, no future—just the experience of now.[4]

BREATH PRACTICES FOR SELF-REGULATION

My friend Bob has been practicing pranayama regularly for twenty-five years because he finds it so helpful for managing his anxiety. Because he wakes up most mornings feeling anxious, he begins his day with conscious breathing, Ujjayi pranayama (a calming breath practice in which you make a sound like the ocean), and other breath practices. These practices help steady him as he gets ready to face the day ahead.

With all pranayama practices, you consciously modify the way you naturally breathe. Doing this focuses your mind, but it can also affect your nervous system and your energy levels. That's how yogic breath practices allow you to calm yourself, energize yourself, or balance yourself. Although many people think that all pranayama practices are relaxing, this is because they consider it only a concentration practice. In reality, some breath practices, such as Skull Shining Breath (Kapalabhati pranayama) and inhalation pausing, are actually stimulating, and others, such as Equal Ratio Breath (Sama Vrtti) and Alternate Nostril Breath (Nadi Sodhana), are actually more "balancing" than relaxing. Understanding how your breath affects your nervous system will help you select which practices you should use when and which practices you might want to avoid. Here's a brief overview.

The part of your nervous system that controls your body's involuntary functions (the functions you don't need to think about) is called the autonomic nervous system. Your autonomic nervous system regulates your essential life functions, including your heartbeat, blood pressure, digestion, and breathing. This same part of your nervous system controls whether you are stressed (in emergencies it triggers a full fight-flight-or-freeze response), very relaxed (in very safe situations it triggers a full rest-and-digest response), or relatively calm and mildly stimulated (for example, when you're involved in an engaging activity).

Of course you cannot instruct your nervous system to lower your blood pressure, speed up your digestion, calm you down, or shake you out of a state of lethargy or sleepiness. But even though you normally breathe without thinking about it, you can consciously change the *way* you breathe. For example, you can intentionally hold your breath, speed up your breath, slow down your breath, make your exhalation longer than your inhalation and vice versa, breathe through one nostril instead of the other, and so on. This is exactly what pranayama consists of: changing the way you breathe! And it is this ability to alter your breathing that gives you the key to your nervous system, providing you with some control over functions that are normally "involuntary."

Here's how it works. With every breath you take, when you inhale, your nervous system stimulates your stress response (fight-flight-or-freeze) to some degree. Then, when you exhale, your nervous system triggers the relaxation response (rest-and-digest) to some degree. When you're breathing naturally, this doesn't change your overall state. However, if you intentionally make your inhalation longer than your exhalation or vice versa for several minutes, this will actually stimulate you or calm you.

When your inhalation is longer than your exhalation, this stimulates your nervous system, triggering a message to your brain that you are in a situation where you need to take action. To ready you for physical and mental action, your brain tells your nervous system to switch you into a modified fight-flight-or-freeze state. So with this breath practice you're indirectly instructing your nervous system to stimulate you and wake you up.

When your exhalation is longer than your inhalation, this quiets your nervous system, increasing the rest-and-digest state while decreasing the fight-flight-or-freeze state. Your brain interprets this to mean you are now safe and don't need to take immediate action. So with this breath practice, you calm your nervous system and mind and lower your stress levels, which will improve your ability to rest, recover, and heal. When you're feeling "stressed," you may notice an improvement after your first few breaths.

When you make your exhalation and inhalation the same length, this has only a very subtle effect on your nervous system. Depending on your current circumstances, this may be slightly stimulating or slightly calming.

Really—how cool is that? Now let's look at some of the pranayama practices and how you might choose which ones to practice when.

Longer inhalations. All pranayama practices that make your inhalations longer than your exhalations are stimulating. These include breath practices where you are actually timing your inhalation, such as when you make your inhalation twice as long as your exhalation or when you do a three-part inhalation (Viloma 2 pranayama) followed by a natural exhalation. In addition, the pause after your inhalation counts is part of your inhalation, so pausing after the inhalation is also stimulating. Finally, there are certain breath practices, such as Skull Shining Breath (Kapalabhati pranayama), that combine quick exhalations with passive inhalations, which naturally make the inhalation longer. You might want to choose this type of practice if you need energizing or are feeling depressed or lethargic. I suggest that you avoid stimulating breath practices when you are feeling hyper, stressed out, anxious, have insomnia, or if they just don't make you feel good.

Longer exhalations. All pranayama practices that make your exhalations longer than your inhalations are calming. These include breath practices where you are actually timing your exhalation, such as when you make your exhalation twice as long as your inhalation or when you do a three-part exhalation (Viloma 1 pranayama) followed by a natural inhalation. In addition, the pause after your exhalation counts as part of your exhalation, so pausing after the exhalation is also calming. Finally, there are certain breath practices, such as Bhramari pranayama, that emphasize the exhalation over the inhalation, which naturally lengthens your exhalations. You might want to choose this type of practice when you are feeling hyper, stressed out, anxious, or have insomnia. I suggest that you avoid calming breath practices only when you're feeling sleepy or lethargic and want to feel more alert or if they just don't make you feel good.

Balanced breathing. All pranayama practices that make your inhalations and exhalations the same length are considered "balancing" in the yoga tradition because, depending on your current state, they will likely be only a bit stimulating or a bit calming. These include breath practices where you are actually timing your inhalations and exhalations to make them the same length, such as Equal Ratio Breath (Sama Vritti). There are also certain breath practices, such as Alternate Nostril Breath, that give equal attention to the inhalations and exhalations, and they naturally tend to make your inhalations and exhalations even. Because these practices don't change your mood and energy levels much, they are good breath practices to choose when you want to settle down and focus, wake yourself up a bit after sleeping, or to simply yoke yourself to the present moment without having a strong effect on your nervous system. I suggest that you avoid balancing practices if they make you feel stressed out or if they just don't make you feel good.

By the way, if you include pausing in your breath practice, for a balanced breath, remember to have equal pausing for both the inhalation and exhalation.

Caution: In this section, I've mentioned some forms of pranayama that are not recommended for beginners, especially in the Iyengar tradition. This is because they can indeed have a very powerful effect on your nervous system. Generally, lengthening your inhalation, lengthening your exhalation, and Bhramari breath are considered fairly safe practices (although you should never let yourself get short of breath and you should never do a breath practice that stresses you out or makes you feel bad). If you are interested in experimenting with pranayama and haven't had any formal instruction, I suggest you study with a trained teacher.

PRANAYAMA BASICS

When and Where to Practice Pranayama

You can practice a session of pranayama on its own, as a prelude to meditation, or as part of a sequence of yoga poses .

When you practice pranayama on its own, you can do it at any time during the day or night. For many years, I practiced exhalation lengthening combined with exhalation pausing to calm myself down when I was stressed, sometimes when I got into bed at night and even in the middle of the night when I woke up and had a hard time falling back to sleep. Just save the stimulating breath practices—if you do them at all—for the daytime.

If you want to combine pranayama with a meditation session, it is traditional to practice pranayama first to steady your mind and then proceed to meditation.

If you want to combine your pranayama practice with your yoga poses, it's traditional to practice pranayama before you begin or after you finish your asana session. Although you can do calming or balancing breath practices either before or after your yoga poses, I suggest that you do stimulating ones—if you do them at all—at the beginning of your practice.

If your goal is to practice pranayama regularly, it's helpful to practice at the same time each day, if possible. So it's a good idea to choose a time when you are usually free. In addition, practicing for short sessions every day is more effective than practicing for a long session less frequently. When you have a routine, eventually your body may tell you it's time to practice, and you may even start to crave your pranayama practice.

However, if the idea of establishing a routine is preventing you from practicing, let it go for now, and simply practice at any time that works for you on a given day. And because we're all dealing with real life, if you do try to establish a routine, you can make exceptions to it on an as-needed basis.

As for where to practice, if your aim is to improve your concentration, prepare for meditating, or regulate your mood, choose any quiet place in your environment that works for you. If there is no quiet place, you can still practice, however. In fact, practicing when there is noise or activity around you trains you to be quiet and calm even during the commotion of everyday life, which is a skill worth cultivating. If your aim is to fall asleep or you are sick or bedbound for any reason, of course you can practice in bed. However, you should otherwise avoid practicing in bed because the lure of sleep might interrupt your practice.

How to Practice Pranayama

Traditionally pranayama is practiced either in a seated position or in a supported Savanasa. If you know you tend to fall asleep in reclined positions, go with a seated position. See Poses for Pranayama and Meditation on page 219 for positions.

Before beginning the pranayama practice, take a few minutes to practice breath awareness as described under How to Practice Breath Awareness on page 18 and observe your natural breath as it is in this moment. Then, at the end of your pranayama practice, practice breath awareness for a few minutes before moving on to your next activity.

How long you should practice depends on your aims and your level of experience. Many people find a short breath practice of even just five minutes is centering. And that amount of time might be a good place to start if you have never practiced before. But if you want to establish a regular practice, Richard Rosen, a longtime pranayama teacher and author of *The Yoga of Breath*, suggests you start by practicing a total of 10 to 12 minutes, with 3 minutes of breath awareness to begin, 5 to 7 minutes of pranayama, and 2 minutes of breath awareness to finish. You can then work up to longer periods of time if desired. And as it happens, 10 to 15 minutes of practice is also the recommended amount of time if you want to trigger the relaxation response with a calming breath practice.

However, because breath practices can have a very strong effect on your nervous system, if you feel anxious, agitated, depressed, or uncomfortable in any way, stop practicing and return to simple breath awareness instead. If that doesn't help—some people feel anxious just from paying attention to their breath—stop your breath practice. Then come into any yoga pose that you find relaxing or comforting, and rest for a few minutes.

As you practice, witness your pranayama practice without judgment just as you would for meditation. If your mind wanders and you lose track of how you're breathing, simply resume the practice without judging yourself. And if any thoughts come into your mind about your ability to practice, simply let them go and return your focus to your breath.

I'm not going to include instructions for practicing the many different forms of pranayama in this chapter because there are entire books, such as *The Yoga of Breath* and *Pranayama beyond the Fundamentals* by Richard Rosen and *Light on Pranayama* by B. K. S. Iyengar, that provide detailed information about the traditional practices. And I myself have already written about some of the simplest and safest ones in *Yoga for Healthy Aging: A Guide to Lifelong Well-Being.*[5]

The following section provides suggestions for a few practices that might be particularly helpful during times of change.

SUGGESTED BREATH PRACTICES

In this section—because, after all, this is not a pranayama book—I'm going to provide instructions for practicing just one basic form of pranayama for each of the three categories, calming, balancing, and stimulating. I consulted with Richard Rosen about my choices because he has so much experience teaching pranayama, and I like his approach to it. For those who already have experience with pranayama, if there is a practice you prefer over the ones I'm suggesting here, please practice whichever ones you prefer.

Calming Breath Practice: Extending the Exhalation (*Vishama Vritti*)

With this practice, you gradually extend your natural exhalation, making it longer and smoother, until you reach your comfortable maximum. Breathe through your nose throughout the practice. If your breath becomes labored or uncomfortable in any way, or you start feeling agitated or panicky, stop and return to your natural breath.

1. After practicing basic breath awareness for a few minutes, without changing your breath, bring your focus to your exhalations. Using the word *om* (not the sound) as a measure, as in 1 om, 2 om, 3 om, count the natural length of your exhalations so you get a sense of what the average length is. After each exhalation, allow your inhalations to come naturally.
2. When you're ready, consciously slow your next exhalation so it is 1 to 3 oms longer than the natural length, keeping it smooth, comfortable, and without any strain. Follow this longer exhalation with a natural inhalation.
3. When you find your comfortable maximum, continue breathing with that extended exhalation and a natural inhalation.
4. If you wish to add exhalation pausing to your breath practice, after lengthening your exhalation, first observe the natural pause that always occurs at the end of each exhalation. Then, when you feel comfortable, allow yourself to "rest" in the pause after the exhalation. If your throat, jaw, tongue, the back of your neck, or other areas feel tense, just notice that. Watch your next inhalation building during this rest and "receive" your inhalation when it feels ready.
5. As time passes and your breath naturally slows, you may find that you can lengthen your exhalation a bit more by adding one or two more oms.
6. At the end of the time you've allocated for pranayama, complete your last extended exhalation and then return to breathing naturally as you practice a few more minutes of breath awareness.

Balancing Breath Practice: Equal Ratio (*Sama Vrtti*)

With this practice, you start by making your inhalations and exhalations the same length. Then, if you wish, you extend both your inhalations and exhalations by the same amount, making them both longer and smoother, until you reach your comfortable maximum. Breathe through your nose throughout the practice. If your breath becomes labored or uncomfortable in any way, or you start feeling agitated or panicky, stop and return to your natural breath.

1. After practicing basic breath awareness for one or two minutes, without changing your breath, count the natural length of your inhalations and exhalations using "om" as a measure, as in "1 om, 2 om, 3 om." Notice which is longer, your inhalation or your exhalation.

2. When you're ready, consciously make both parts of your breath last the same number of oms by making the longer part of your breath the same number of oms as the shorter part. For example, if your inhalation is naturally around 5 oms while your exhalation is around 7 oms, you would make both your inhalation and exhalation 5 oms long. Practice this equal breath for three to four rounds.

3. If you're comfortable with the current length of your inhalations and exhalations, simply keep practicing this equal breath for your entire session. Or, if you'd like to lengthen both your inhalation and exhalation, at this point, add one more om onto both parts of your breath. Practice with the longer length for three to four rounds. (You can keep repeating this process of lengthening both your inhalation and exhalation by one om after every three or four rounds until you reach your comfortable maximum.)

4. At the end of the time you've allocated for pranayama, complete your last exhalation and then return to breathing naturally as you practice a few more minutes of breath awareness.

Stimulating Breath Practice: Skull Shining Breath (*Kapalabhati*)

Skull Shining Breath is an energizing breath practice that makes you more present and alert, especially when you're feeling sleepy or sluggish. Typically in your everyday breath your exhalation is longer than your inhalation. With Skull Shining Breath you make your exhalation short and fast by quickly contracting your abdominal muscles towards your spine as you breathe out. Then you follow that quick exhalation with a slightly slower rebound inhalation. The rapid breathing and strong abdominal contractions mildly stimulate your fight-flight-or-freeze response.

For those of you who have no previous experience with this practice, Richard Rosen recommends learning the practice in a reclined position with your fingertips on your lower abdomen to help you learn how to contract your muscles on your exhalation. Breathe through your nose throughout the practice. If you start feeling agitated, panicky, or uncomfortable in any way, stop and return to your natural breath.

Here's the basic approach:

1. With your fingertips placed lightly on your lower belly, breathe normally and observe your natural breath for a few minutes. Notice how as you exhale your lower belly firms to help push your breath out of your lungs.
2. When you're ready to take your first Skull Shining Breath, begin with a moderate inhalation. Next, quickly contract your lower belly to push your exhalation out of your lungs and through your nose with a "whoosh" sound. Then, just as quickly, relax your lower belly and passively allow your next inhalation to flow into your lungs.
3. Take a natural breath and then repeat the Skull Shining Breath.
4. Continue alternating between a natural breath and a Skull Shining Breath a few more times.
5. Now check in with yourself. Are you feeling comfortable or uncomfortable? Stimulated, exhilarated, or faint? If that's enough for you, return to your natural breath. If you're doing fine, continue practicing Skull Shining Breath for a total of ten to twelve times. This is one round.
6. Breathe naturally for 30 seconds to 1 minute and see if another round is possible. If so, practice another round of 10 to 12 Skull Shining Breaths, followed by another 30-second to 1-minute rest.
7. If you're still up for it, repeat a round of Skull Shining Breath for a total of 3 rounds.
8. Return to your natural breath and practice simple breath awareness, observing the effects of the breath practices on your energy levels and mood.

This practice will help you get accustomed to this way of breathing, and after a few weeks, you may feel ready to advance in your practice. I suggest that you consult with an experienced teacher for the next phase.

Meditation

As for where the mind wanders to: well, lots of places, obviously, but studies have shown that these places are usually in the past or the future; you may ponder recent events or distant, strong memories; you may dread upcoming events or eagerly anticipate them; you may strategize about how to head off some looming crisis or fantasize about romancing the attractive person in the cubicle next to yours. What you're generally not doing when your mind is wandering is directly experiencing the present moment.

—Robert Wright, *Why Buddhism Is True*

Although there are many different forms of meditation, all forms train you to be present. Whatever you choose to meditate on—your breath, a mantra, the sensations in your body, the sounds in the room—you are focusing on something that is taking place in the here and now. And when you notice your mind wandering, you bring it back to the present, again and again. Although you're not present the entire time you meditate, repeating this process of bringing your mind back to your object of meditation trains you to notice when you're not present in your everyday life and to then return your focus to the present.

ACCEPTING IMPERMANENCE

Being present during meditation in turn teaches you to be more comfortable with impermanence and change. As you notice how your thoughts come and go, how your breath changes from moment to moment, how various sounds arise and then fall away (a car drives by, a breeze rustles the bamboo leaves, a squirrel chitters briefly in a nearby tree, a child laughs in the distance), all these things remind you over and over that change is intrinsic to our life here on earth. The yoga and mindfulness meditation teacher Jill Satterfield says:

By watching my mind for so many years now, I've befriended impermanence and change. Stability in anything except awareness has gone off the wish list, which has made my life more full of ease. This is the sanity and ease of not knowing: being comfortable—not always liking, but being comfortable—with change.[6]

When I meditate in the morning in the winter, I practice in front of a window, and I can sense the sun rising through my closed eyes. This allows me to experience change on a visceral level, as the earth revolves on its axis, moving us all through day and night, day and night.

QUIETING YOUR MIND

As you train yourself to be present, meditating can bring you feelings of peace and contentment because the practice quiets your mind. After several minutes of meditation, your nervous system triggers the relaxation response, which lowers your stress levels. This in turn slows down your thoughts and may even change the types of thoughts you're having. When you're more relaxed, your repertoire of thoughts expands to include more compassionate and altruistic thoughts than you typically have when you're stressed. Eventually, if you meditate long enough, you may have the experience where your mind quiets so much you reach a state where your thoughts cease entirely.

OBSERVING YOUR THOUGHTS

Meditation also trains you to notice your thoughts and to observe what you tend to think about. Observing your thought patterns can be helpful when you want to learn about which thoughts you are having that are untrue or that are not serving you well (see Accepting Your Thoughts and Feelings on page 231). Dr. Scott Lauzé explains it like this:

Repeating this process of noticing, taking note, and then letting go and returning to the present moment allows us to know ourselves better. We get on to ourselves. We can notice that there are places our mind likes to go habitually, and how that makes us feel. . . . We also learn to see that our minds frequently send us down thought paths that are not grounded in the reality of the present moment, and our minds also send us thoughts that are "fake news."[7]

The moment that you notice you are thinking or reacting automatically—the precious pause—is the time you have for changing those reactions and thought patterns, both during meditation and in your daily life. And as you move your focus away from distracting thoughts and emotions during meditation, you are learning to let go of them.

However, although all types of meditation bring you into the present and enable you to cultivate equanimity and reduce stress, the three basic types actually have different aims, provide different in-the-moment experiences, and have different long-term effects. So the following section provides an overview of the differences and similarities for the three types. You can then choose the type that's right for you or even switch to a new type if you're ready for a change.

TYPES OF MEDITATION

In some yoga traditions, only one type of meditation is recommended, typically concentration meditation. And you are advised to find a single way of practicing that type of meditation and to stick with it. In Buddhism, however, it's common to practice concentration meditation at the beginning of a meditation session and then move into mindfulness meditation. And in some Tantra Yoga traditions the view is that any type of meditation that works for you is the best one for you and that changing the way you meditate when you feel stuck in a rut can help you deepen your practice. So for this book I'm providing information about how to practice all three basic types. (In my research, I've seen these types labeled and categorized in several different ways, so bear with me if I use different categories than the ones you're used to.)

Concentration Meditation

The first type of meditation is the classic yoga technique called concentration meditation, focused attention, or one-pointed awareness—among other names. It consists of concentrating on a single object of meditation (your breath, a mantra, an image, and so on) and, when your attention wanders, bringing your awareness back to the object. The aim for this type of meditation is to quiet the mind, eventually stopping all thoughts, emotions, and sensations (restricting the movements of consciousness). Because this technique is so quieting for the mind, it is sometimes called serenity or tranquility meditation.

If you are following the eightfold path described in the Yoga Sutras, this technique is what will enable you to reach a state of samadhi, meditative absorption. In the Tantra Yoga tradition, this meditation technique is one of many ways to unite with the universal consciousness. And Buddhism uses concentration meditation to steady the mind before practicing mindfulness meditation.

Concentration meditation cultivates your ability to be in the present moment—you return your focus repeatedly to the here and now, away from thoughts or feelings about the past or future. Regularly quieting your mind and training yourself to focus on the present help you to cultivate equanimity through the ups and downs of your everyday life. And scientific studies have shown that this type of meditation sharpens your ability to focus.

Training the Mind and Heart

The second type of meditation focuses on cultivating a particular feeling, such as compassion, gratitude, joy, or relaxation, or on cultivating a particular mental state. The aim for these practices is to affect the way you feel or think in the moment and also to have a lasting effect that shows up in your everyday life. The most common are loving-kindness meditations, gratitude practices, and relaxation practices. For people who find that sitting alone with their thoughts sends them into a downward spiral (which can be dangerous for those with depression and anxiety), one of these highly structured and/or guided meditations might be engaging enough to keep you grounded in the here and now.

Tantra Yoga uses this type of meditation to allow you to commune with different aspects of the universal consciousness. For example, by meditating on joy, delight, or satisfaction you can access the experience of *ananda* (bliss), which Christopher Wallis defines as "a state of absolute contentment, acceptance, and quiet yet sublime joy: the peace that passeth all understanding."[8]

This type of meditation, like basic concentration meditation, cultivates your ability to be in the present moment because you return your focus repeatedly to the here and now, away from thoughts or feelings about the past or future. But the long-term effects of these practices differ, depending on which one you practice. For example, a loving-kindness meditation can help reduce or remove violent feelings toward others, such as hatred and desire for revenge. And scientists have discovered that it strengthens regions of your brain that are associated with "socially driven emotions," such as empathy. See Training the Mind and Heart on page 210 for more information.

Mindfulness Meditation

This third type of meditation is the "open-monitoring" technique that was originally taught by Siddhārtha Gautama, the Buddha. It consists of nonjudgmentally observing your thoughts, emotions, and physical sensations. Rather than "restricting" the movements of your consciousness, you cultivate awareness of them.

The aim for this type of practice is to learn to see reality as it is—impermanent and ever changing—and to make peace with this reality. It is also intended to allow you to observe how your mind works, to understand that your thoughts and feelings do not define who you are, and to "liberate" you from the suffering caused by distressing mind-states such as anger, fear, greed, jealousy, and hatred.

Mindfulness meditation cultivates your ability to be in the present moment because you maintain your focus on thoughts, feelings, and sensations in the present rather than allowing your mind to wander to the past or future. This is a mental skill you can take into your everyday life to make you less reactive in challenging situations and to help improve your relationships with others. Scientific studies have shown that this type of meditation caused changes in areas of the brain associated with understanding the mental states of others.

In some yoga traditions, such as Tantra and Hatha, this form of meditation, as well as many other forms, is used to unite with the universal consciousness. And Tantra Yoga specifically uses mindfulness meditation practices to allow you to become aware of the unchanging, eternal witness to all your experiences.

If you can't decide which type of meditation to practice, just pick something that appeals to you. If that sounds flaky, consider that some of the oldest advice on meditation, sutra I.39 of the Yoga Sutras, simply says that you can achieve steadiness meditating on anything you like.

> Or [steadiness of the mind is attained] from meditation upon anything of one's inclination.[9]

It's also okay to experiment. In *Meditation for the Love of It* Sally Kempton says that after you become familiar with a technique, it should feel natural.[10] So if after several days of practice you feel you still have to work very hard, that could mean that's the wrong technique for you. Try something else and see how that goes.

MEDITATION BASICS

This section provides instructions that apply to all forms of meditation. This is followed by specific instructions for practicing the three different types I described earlier.

Before I get started, however, for those who are not already meditating, you should know that while meditation is a very powerful technique for being present and for making peace with change, the practice is not necessarily for everyone. If you are experiencing anxiety or depression, for example, it actually could worsen your condition. Dr. Lynn Somerstein, who is both a yoga therapist and a psychoanalyst, had this to say about meditating when you have depression:

> Meditation itself can turn on you and become a litany of self-blame and despair. You might think you're meditating and helping yourself, but you're not; you're ruminating, digging yourself into a deeper and deeper hole. So the biggest contraindication to meditating is severe unregulated depression, and this must be respected because the rumination picks up steam and can drive you into the depths.[11]

Dr. Scott Lauzé says the same is true for people with untreated psychotic disorders and significant trauma (or PTSD) that has not already been worked through in therapy. He explains that for both these conditions, the emotions that come up with inward looking and opening the mind can be "overwhelming, destabilizing, and scary."[12] It's a good idea if you are suffering from any of these conditions to check in with a mental health professional before starting a practice.

In general, I think it makes sense that if you find a certain practice is depressing, agitating, or causes anxiety, or that it sends you into a downward spiral, you should choose practices that are active and less inward-focused for the time being. Most people find that practicing yoga poses mindfully can be very helpful because the practice takes you out of your mind and into your body (see Coping Skill 5: Taking a Break with a Mindful Asana Practice on page 40). Of course, if you already have longtime experience with meditation, it can be safe to meditate if you conclude that practicing helps you.

When and Where to Practice

Traditionally, meditators practice at times of "transition," such as at the beginning or end of the day, or even at midday. But if your intuition—or your schedule—suggests a different time, practice when it's best for you.

If your goal is to meditate regularly, it's helpful to meditate at the same time each day, if possible. So it's a good idea to choose a time when you are usually free. In addition, practicing for short sessions every day is more effective for establishing a routine than practicing a long session less frequently. When you have a routine, eventually your body may tell you it's time to practice, and you may even start to crave your meditation practice.

However, if the idea of establishing a routine is preventing you from practicing, let it go for now and simply practice at any time that works for you on a given day. And because we're all dealing with real life, if you do try to establish a routine, you can make exceptions to it on an as-needed basis.

If you want to combine your meditation practice with a sequence of yoga poses, it's traditional to practice either before or after your asana practice. If you're also combining pranayama with your meditation practice, practice your pranayama before you meditate.

As for where to practice, if you can, choose a quiet place anywhere in your environment that works for you. However, if there is no quiet place, you can still practice. In fact, meditating when there is noise or activity around you trains you to be quiet and calm even during the commotion of everyday life, which is a skill worth cultivating. If your aim is to fall asleep or you are sick or bedbound for any reason, of course you can practice in bed. However, you should otherwise avoid practicing in bed because the lure of sleep might interrupt your practice.

While it is good to stay flexible about where you meditate, an advantage to meditating in the same place every day with the same setup or on the same chair is that this habit can condition you to settle more quickly into a quiet mind.

How to Practice Meditation

You don't always need to meditate in a special position or in a special way—I've been known to meditate to the sound of the waves while lying on the sand at the beach or to the sounds of nature in a forest while sitting on a rock. The only essential element for practicing all types of meditation is to refrain from making judgments as you practice, which I will describe next. For your regular at-home meditation practice, however, putting in the extra time to set yourself up in a comfortable position, gradually working your way up to longer practices, and marking the transitions into and out of practice can help you settle in more quickly and reach deeper states of meditation. The following list provides some basic suggestions for how to practice:

Witnessing without judgment. This practice helps to quiet your mind and allows you to focus on your meditation. So as you meditate, maintain a neutral approach to your meditation experience and witness all your thoughts and feelings without evaluating them. When you notice your mind wandering, let go of the distracting thoughts and emotions, and simply resume meditating again without judging yourself. And if any thoughts come into your mind about your ability to practice, let those go too.

If you have a hard time letting go of thoughts and emotions by just resuming meditation, there are several different techniques you can use to actively let go. See Letting Go on page 234 for information about letting go of thoughts and emotions both during meditation and in everyday life.

Meditation positions. For positions to meditate in, you actually have a number of options. Although we typically see meditation being practiced in a seated pose with closed eyes, you can practice lying down or even standing as well. (See Poses for Pranayama and Meditation on page 219 for poses to choose from). And it is actually traditional to practice meditation either with open or closed eyes. So, if closing your eyes in meditation causes agitation or brooding, keep your eyes open but with a soft focus. Gaze downward instead of straight out at the world. Try opening your eyes fully (full-moon eyes), one half (half-moon eyes), or one quarter (new-moon eyes), and see what works best for you.

Timing. How long you should practice depends on what your aim is. Many people find that a short meditation practice of even just five minutes is "centering." But if you want to really quiet your mind—or study it in depth with mindfulness meditation—consider gradually working your way toward longer practices. When you're practicing concentration meditation, it takes ten to fifteen minutes for the relaxation response to take full effect; an even longer practice (one or more hours) can lead you into deeper states of meditation, which you can learn about in *Meditation for the Love of It* by Sally Kempton.

That being said, if meditating ever makes you feel anxious, agitated, depressed, or in a downward mental spiral, stop practicing, even before your time is up. Then come into any yoga pose that you do find relaxing or comforting, and rest for a few minutes.

Marking the transitions. Before you meditate, if you like, you can perform a short ritual to mark the transition to your practice. This can help you slow down and move into a more receptive frame of mind for your meditation. What you do is up to you—light a candle, burn some incense, take a moment to express gratitude in whatever fashion you like, and so on. Then, when you end your session, you can perform a second ritual to ease your transition back into everyday life.

HOW TO PRACTICE CONCENTRATION MEDITATION

With this form of meditation, choosing a mental focus for your meditation session is key. You have a large number of choices, however, and you can experiment to see what works best for you.

Breath

Your breath is a particularly good mental focus for cultivating steadiness of mind and for improving your ability to focus. When you focus your attention on your breath, even though you don't intend to change it, just bringing your awareness to it tends to slow it down and make it more even. And because the way you breathe affects your stress-hormone levels—one of which, noradrenaline, affects your ability to focus— breathing more slowly and evenly can take you to a "sweet spot" where your thinking is clearer and your ability to focus improves.

There are many different ways to focus on your breath, and you can choose whichever works best for you. See Coping Skill 1: Centering Yourself with Breath

Awareness on page 17 for some suggestions. In some yoga traditions, focusing on the spaces between your breaths—the pauses at the ends of your inhalations and the ends of your exhalations—without changing their length allows you to experience a point of stillness. And this central still point is considered an "open door into the heart of the universe."[13]

But meditating on your breath isn't for everyone. Some people become anxious about their breathing when they focus on it, and others may have respiratory problems or even a common cold that make it unpleasant to focus on their breath. In these situations, using a mantra or visual image might be a better choice. For me, I've found that meditating on my breath isn't enough to engage my mind, so I combine a mantra practice with awareness of my breath.

Visual Images

As a mental focus, you can gaze with open eyes on a single object, such as a candle flame, a star in the sky, or a single point in front of you. Practicing with eyes fixed on an object is called *trataka*. Some people find it easier to focus on an external image than on something internal. If you want to practice with eyes closed, you can just picture an object in your mind's eye. My friend yoga teacher Patrice Priya Wagner uses a sculpture on her mantelpiece in just this way. She says that "Being a very visual person, I found that an image would stick in my mind to keep out random thoughts more easily than other points of focus."[14]

Sound

For a concentration practice, you can focus on a single sound that repeats, such as the ringing of a bell or the sound of waves breaking on the seashore. This experience can be hard to arrange, but I think it's something to take advantage of when it's available. The most beautiful meditation experience I ever had was a Tibetan gong meditation. Observing the sounds arise and then fade away can teach you about impermanence.

Mantras

Mantras are phrases that you either recite out loud or to yourself. If you wish, you can coordinate the recitation with your breath. Simply inhale and then repeat the mantra on your exhalation.

Mantras can be in the traditional language of yoga, Sanskrit, or in any other language you choose. Because different mantras have different meanings, you should choose them with care. While some are just intended to quiet the mind and bring feelings of peace, others are intended to cultivate a particular emotion or frame of mind. I'll suggest a few here for cultivating peace of mind. See Training the Mind and Heart below for some others.

Some traditional Sanskrit mantras for cultivating peace of mind include:

- SO HUM: The "breathing mantra" that sounds like your inhalation and exhalation. It means "I am that." "That" is the universe so you are identifying yourself with the universe.
- OM: The divine in the form of sound.
- OM SHANTI: An invocation of peace.
- SHANTI, SHANTI, SHANTI or OM SHANTI, SHANTI, SHANTI: Peace from suffering caused by the divine, by the material world, and from self-inflicted suffering.

You can also choose a phrase in any language that has meaning to you. When she was the caregiver for both her elderly parents and needed a mantra to keep her steady through crisis after crisis, Elissa C. Rosenthal, a yoga teacher and registered occupational therapist, chose a mantra in the language of her spiritual heritage, Hebrew. She recited "HINENI. CHAZAK. HAR." This translates to "Here I am. Strong. A Mountain." Elissa now says, "This has become my go-to mantra when my faith in my ability to endure falters."[15]

TRAINING THE MIND AND HEART

Meditations that train the mind and heart are all forms of concentration meditation, so you practice them the same way as basic concentration meditation (described earlier). You choose one "object" to focus on during your meditation, whether it's a feeling, a wish, an idea, or an image, and when you notice your mind wandering, simply bring it back to the focus you chose.

What's different about these types of meditations is that they are not intended just to quiet your mind. Instead, they are designed to help you cultivate a particular feeling or mental/emotional skill. The following sections provide information about some of the most common meditations for training the mind and heart, describing how they differ and what their long-lasting effects might be.

Loving-Kindness (*Maitri*) Meditations

Loving-kindness meditations are formal, scripted practices in which you send love and compassion to a range of people about whom you feel differently, including yourself. Cultivating loving-kindness in your meditation can help reduce or remove negative feelings toward others, such as hatred and desire for revenge. A study on brain morphology and three types of meditation found that Maitri meditation caused strengthening of regions in the brain that are associated with "socially driven emotions," such as empathy. You can find loving-kindness meditations in many books on meditation as well as online.

Universal Kindness

If you want to focus on a single person or on cultivating a single emotional skill, rather than practicing the full loving-kindness meditation, you can meditate on any one of the following: unconditional friendship (*maitri*), compassion (*karuna*), sympathetic joy (*mudita*), equanimity (*upeksha*). You can also focus just on forgiveness (*kshama*). These are all described in chapter 8 in the section Letting Go. And for the meditation, you can just focus on any person or group, on yourself, or even just on "all beings."

Love

You can meditate on your love for someone as a way to reconnect to that feeling, to feel connected to someone who died or whom you can't see, or to help let go of anger toward someone you care about. See Witness Grief with a Concentration Meditation on page 155 for details.

Gratitude Meditations

Meditations on gratitude include both formal and informal practices in which you express your gratitude for things you appreciate, both small and large, in your life. Cultivating gratitude in your meditation can help reduce or remove negative feelings, such as unhappiness and dissatisfaction, and can improve your sense of well-being. Science tells us that a gratitude practice can produce both dopamine and serotonin, and serotonin is, among other things, a mood stabilizer, reducing depression and anxiety. The simplest way to practice this is to simply focus on a person or thing that you are grateful for and to mentally express your gratitude. But you can also find guided gratitude meditations.

Relaxation Meditation

This category includes the formal practice of yoga nidra as well as other meditations in which you are guided by a teacher or self-guided with instructions designed to make you feel relaxed, reduce stress, fall asleep, and so on. Cultivating relaxation quiets your nervous system and reduces the levels of stress hormones in the body. Lasting effects can include lower baseline stress levels, improved sleep, a less reactive nervous system, reduced anxiety, and healing from trauma.

Sensual Meditations

Tantra Yoga has a tradition of meditations in which you immerse yourself in a sensory experience. This practice enables you to experience the world directly—smelling, tasting, hearing, feeling, and seeing—without the mental constructs that prevent you from being fully present with the world around you. You can choose almost any type of object to become absorbed in. You could savor a peach or a cup of coffee. You could immerse yourself in a work of art, such as music or a painting. You could engage your senses by appreciating a flower or a tree.

Christopher Wallis says that in non-dual Saiva Tantra this is called "feeding the goddesses of the senses." And when you feed the goddesses, they will

> reward you by suffusing your awareness with aesthetic rapture (*chanakara*), increasing your capacity to experience beauty. The whole world becomes more vivid and real, more radiantly lovely, more full of life-energy.[16]

Other Mental States

Many Tantric meditations are designed to allow you to experience different aspects of the universal consciousness. You might meditate on joy, delight, or satisfaction. You might fill yourself with light, love, or spaciousness. You might meditate on complete darkness or emptiness. It is said that these experiences can help you reach a true understanding of the nature of universal consciousness, the supreme reality. The Vijnana Bhairava, a traditional Tantra text, includes many of these meditations, and you can find others in modern books on yoga meditation.

HOW TO PRACTICE MINDFULNESS MEDITATION

To be clear, in this type of meditation, instead of focusing on a mantra or the breath for the whole time, you spend some time simply sitting in a space of quiet openness, with a willingness to see whatever needs to be seen, to feel whatever wants to be felt, neither seeking nor pushing away thoughts but simply watching nonjudgmentally whatever arises and subsides.

—Christopher D. Wallis, *Tantra Illuminated*

Mindfulness meditation is intended to teach you to be present with whatever arises. So while for concentration meditation you turn your attention *away* from anything except your object of meditation, in mindfulness meditation you turn your attention *toward* what is arising in the present moment. This includes both what is arising within you—physical sensations, emotions, thoughts—as well as what is occurring in the environment around you, such as sounds or smells.

The result is that mindfulness meditation is not necessarily as quieting as a concentration practice because you are sometimes exploring difficult things, such as an uncomfortable emotion or a sound that normally irritates you. However, because the practice trains you to fully engage with what's happening in the present, it can teach you to be more present in your everyday life with whatever challenges arise. As Tara Brach explained, "The purpose of mindfulness meditation is to become mindful throughout all parts of our life, so that we're awake, present and openhearted in everything we do."[17]

Author and teacher of mindfulness meditation and yoga Charlotte Bell says that the equanimity she maintained through her experience with breast cancer was a "testament" to twenty-eight years of mindfulness practice.

While it was not the diagnosis I had hoped for, my mind never descended into "why me?" or "poor me" or "what did I do to deserve this?" or any such machinations. I saw the diagnosis simply as a new context for me.[18]

Although we can't necessarily expect the same results from a regular mindfulness meditation that Charlotte had—and you should not feel ashamed if you don't react to a cancer diagnosis or other traumatic news with the equanimity that she did—I thought her story was so inspiring that I wanted to share it with you. And this story does illustrate so powerfully the potential that a long-term mindfulness meditation practice has to help us cope during times of change.

Typically you start a mindfulness practice with a few minutes of concentration meditation to settle your mind. You can then open your awareness to what's happening within you, such as your thoughts, emotions, or physical sensations, or what's happening outside you, such as external sounds, or both.

Mindfulness is a special kind of observation, however. It means seeing things in a new way. So whatever you turn your awareness to, rather than just "being in the moment," set an intention to do two things.

1. **Notice what is happening.** This means pausing long enough to recognize whatever is actually occurring and naming it even.
2. **Accept what is happening.** This means simply allowing whatever is happening in the present to occur, and not trying to push away any of the sensations, emotions, or thoughts you experience, even uncomfortable or painful ones.

Countless books have been written just about how to practice mindfulness meditation, so I'll briefly outline just a few of the specific practices that I've learned about that I think you might find especially useful during times of change.

Sounds

Many practitioners, including me, find that hearing meditation is a really helpful way to begin daily practice. Hearing meditation helps ground us in time and space. Relaxing into the landscape of changing sounds is relatively effortless. Also, it's very easy to listen to sound and not take it personally.

—Charlotte Bell

You can use your mindfulness practice to be fully present with the environment around you through your sense of hearing. This practice can help settle you in the present moment, and it allows you to sense how connected you are to the "external" world.

Because you're not focusing on yourself—and you can hear sounds in the environment coming from places you can't even see—this practice can really take you out of your head. And Charlotte Bell says that hearing meditations teach you to relax not only into your sense of hearing but also into other sensations that arise. It's a common way to start a mindfulness practice, but you could also use it as a focus for your entire practice.

You can practice inside a room or out in nature. Start by noticing the sounds closest to you and gradually move outward to sounds you detect in the distance. Notice judgments you make about them, which you like and which you dislike. Let go and listen to the sounds as sounds. Notice how they arise and fall—a lesson in impermanence.

Physical Sensations

> Mindfulness of the body is one of the foundations of mindfulness practice. We experience literally everything through our senses. We even experience our thoughts, mental states, and emotions as sensations in our bodies. So the ability to anchor our awareness in our bodies is very important.
> —Charlotte Bell

Even when your mind is in the past or the future, your pulsing, breathing body is always in the present. That's why focusing on your physical sensations in your meditation—taking your awareness out of your head and into your body—is one of the foundations of mindfulness meditation. This type of meditation can be especially helpful if you're someone with an especially busy mind. And it's a practice you can turn to in daily life when you notice yourself getting caught up in a whirlwind of regrets about the past or worries about the future.

To focus on your physical sensations, you can use both your external sense of touch to feel what is touching your skin as well as your internal senses of interoception and proprioception (described under Coping Skill 5: Taking a Break with a Mindful Asana Practice in chapter 2) to feel what's going on inside your body. One way to practice is to gradually scan your body, from your toes to the crown of your head, noticing, without judgment, whatever you feel. Notice any movements, however minor. Is there a feeling of comfort, discomfort, or even pain? Do you sense relaxation or tension? Itching or tingling? Coolness or warmth?

You can also focus on a single area of your body that is calling out for attention, perhaps because there is discomfort there or even pain. Because sensations of discomfort and pain typically move in waves, arising and then receding, this practice can teach you about impermanence in a very visceral way. For physical pain, exploring the sensations of pain in a nonjudgmental way can even reduce the intensity of the pain. However, Charlotte Bell cautions that it's essential not to bring your awareness to pain with the intention of making the pain go away, but simply to explore it with curiosity and openness. In addition, respect your intuition about whether the time is right for you to do this practice. And if you *are* practicing and notice yourself tightening up or the pain gets more intense, this could be a sign it's best to focus elsewhere instead. In general, if you want to work with chronic pain in your meditation, it is best to get guidance from an expert.

Emotions

> By creating an environment of permission within, we release the expectation that painful states of mind like anger or depression or fear will consume us. They can arise and we can let them go. It's a practice—of not holding on, of choosing *not* to identify, *not* to think, *This is who I am. This is who I will always be.*
>
> —Sharon Salzberg, *Real Change*

In chapters 4 and 5 I discussed how there may be times when you realize that you need to move through or let go of a painful emotion. One way to do this is by focusing on the emotion itself in your meditation, as opposed to the incident that is causing the emotion. When you observe the emotion nonjudgmentally as a set of sensations, the simple act of paying attention to it may actually reduce the intensity of the emotion so you're no longer overwhelmed by it. As Sally Kempton says:

> It is one of the most important things you can teach yourself through meditation: how to hold strong feelings in Awareness and how to allow Awareness to dissolve them. Once you know how to do it, you'll no longer fear your own feelings.[19]

To practice, start by bringing to mind the thought or situation that is provoking the emotion, whether it's sadness, fear, shame, anger, or something else. Then, as the emotion associated with the story arises within you, move your awareness away from the story to the sensations caused by the emotion itself. Whatever you are feeling, explore it nonjudgmentally. Where do you feel it in your body and what do you feel there? Charlotte Bell says that if you observe the emotion as a set of sensations that "arise, intensify, decrease, dissolve, or reappear," it can help you see that the nature of an emotion is that it is a "passing phenomenon."[20]

If the emotion does not decrease in intensity as you bring awareness to it, you can intentionally let it go. Inhale and bring your awareness to the emotion and then release it as you exhale.

If at any time this practice becomes too much for you, simply return to the concentration meditation you used to start your practice.

Thoughts

> This practice shows us where we are spending our mental energy. What are the thoughts that are most persistent for us? What emotions or mental states do these persistent thoughts evoke? This practice can help us to choose which thoughts are productive and worth pursuing, and which are not productive and therefore worthy of letting go.
>
> —Charlotte Bell

You can use your mindfulness practice to be present with the thoughts you're having as you meditate. This will develop your ability to notice that thoughts are always arising and falling away in your mind throughout your waking hours—your internal monologue, as it is often called. It can also help you realize that just because you're having a thought doesn't mean that it's true (see Accepting Your Thoughts and Feelings on page 231 for more information about this). For example, for a long time, I noticed that while I was meditating I always had the same panicky thought: "I'll never make it through this whole session!" I eventually realized that sitting alone with my thoughts reminded me of having insomnia and being awake in the middle of the night with thoughts racing through my mind—morning seemed like it would never come. But the truth was I always did make it through my meditation sessions—as well as my insomnia attacks—and eventually I just had to laugh when I noticed that same old thought arising.

To practice being present with your thoughts, you can just set an intention to notice each time you have a thought, first by recognizing it and then by accepting it, no matter what kind of thought it is. But if you want to learn about your habitual thought patterns, a very useful technique is to label your thoughts. Labeling your thoughts helps you learn whether you typically ruminate about the past, worry about the future, make negative judgments about the present or about yourself, and so on. And learning what your unhelpful—or untrue—thought patterns are is the first step toward letting go of them. As mindfulness teacher Sharon Salzberg says in *Real Change*:

> We can retrain our whole mental attitude by first learning to recognize these patterns, and perhaps even calmly naming them: "Oh, here is the pattern of thinking, Everything is wrong, the pattern of thinking, I'm a failure, the pattern of thinking, Nothing will ever change." Once we recognize them, we can remind ourselves these are just visiting, they are not essentially who we are, we could not stop them from visiting, but we can let them go.[21]

You can use whatever labels you wish, probably based on what you initially observe as "untrue" or "unhelpful." For example, I have a "panicking too soon" label for plans I start making for things that might not even happen.

After you have experience observing your thought patterns during meditation, you will develop the ability to notice that same habitual thinking in your daily life. And when you notice you're being caught up in those same old patterns, you then have the possibility of letting go of those thoughts or even cultivating opposite thoughts (see Letting Go on page 234 for more information).

Daily Life

The purpose of mindfulness meditation is to teach you to be more present in your everyday life, not just when you meditate. And intentionally practicing this technique in your everyday life, for example, when you're brushing your teeth or drinking your morning cup of tea or coffee, enables you to integrate what you've learned about mindfulness into real-world situations. You'll then be able to call on these skills during difficult situations when they might be of great benefit to you. In addition, practicing mindfulness in your daily life is a beautiful way to experience your aliveness. As Christopher Wallis says: "even mundane daily actions like washing the dishes and walking the dog are opportunities for experiencing the joy that flows naturally from the holistic awareness of being in full Presence."[22]

Making mindfulness in daily life a regular practice can be life changing because, as Charlotte Bell told me, "This daily practice can turn into a jumping-off point for developing a habit of mindfulness in the rest of our lives."[23] She recommends that you pick one simple activity that you do every day—washing the dishes, taking a walk, making your bed, drinking your morning cup of tea or coffee—and commit to practicing it mindfully each day. For whatever activity you choose, give your full attention to it, acknowledging and accepting all the sensations you experience during the activity as well as the thoughts and emotions you have in response to them. For example, if you are drinking a cup of tea, through each step in the process—holding the cup, lifting the cup, touching the cup to your lips, having the tea in your mouth, swallowing the tea, lowering the cup and setting it down—what do you see, smell, taste, hear, and feel? And do any of your sense impressions trigger specific thoughts or emotions? After that, take a moment to notice whether you feel any aftereffects from your tea-drinking experience. Then observe the sensations, thoughts, and emotions that prompt you to take another sip of tea or to do something else instead.

Eventually after practicing this way you'll be ready to turn your full attention to other activities in your everyday life as well.

Poses for Pranayama and Meditation

Because we typically use the same seated and reclined positions for both pranayama and meditation, I'm describing the seated and reclined positions for both in this section. For meditation, I'm also including the option of meditating standing up in case that's something you'd like to try. For all positions, it's important to be comfortable. So if needed, make any necessary adjustments, even while you're in the pose. Just be careful to move slowly and carefully so your movements don't disturb your quiet mind.

SEATED POSITIONS

If you want to practice in a seated position, you can sit in any comfortable, stable seated pose, such as Easy Sitting pose, Hero pose, or even Half or Full Lotus pose

(Ardha Padmasana or Padmasana). Being comfortable is essential because pain or discomfort will distract you, so be honest with yourself about how long you can stay comfortably in the pose you choose. If you feel like having support for your back would make you more comfortable or stable, you can sit with your pelvis and upper back touching a wall.

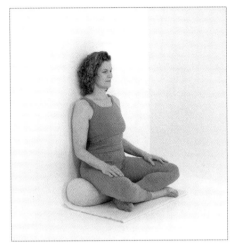

You can also practice sitting on a chair.

For all seated positions, pay attention to your posture after you sit down and throughout your practice. While maintaining the natural curves of your spine, keep your spine long and your head directly over the top of it. And keep your chest open by widening your collarbones away from each other and firming your shoulder blades against your back.

These adjustments may help you breathe more easily (and allow the prana to flow) and may also keep your back happier.

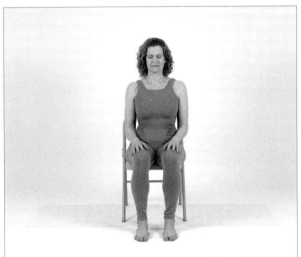

If you want to sit on the floor and don't already have experience with sitting in a yoga pose with good posture for longer periods, Richard Rosen recommends you practice in Easy Sitting pose with your back against the wall or some other flat surface. Sit on a support, such as a folded blanket, to help keep your pelvis in a neutral position, and place a rolled-up towel in the curve of your lower back. This way you can feel your shoulder blades pressing against the wall while you maintain the natural curves of your spine.

For pranayama, place your hands on your thighs, palms down. If this hand position makes your shoulders tense, try placing a folded blanket on your lap to support your hands. For meditation, you can use the same hand position, or if you practice mudras, whatever mudra is appropriate for your practice.

If the seated position you chose is asymmetrical, such as Easy Sitting pose or Half Lotus, be sure to alternate the cross of your legs from day to day.

RECLINED POSITIONS

For pranayama, if you want to practice in a reclined position, choose a supported version of Savasana where your torso is higher than your pelvis and legs and your head is higher than your torso. Although you could use the same version of Supported Savasana that you use for relaxation, typically the setup for pranayama has less support than ver-

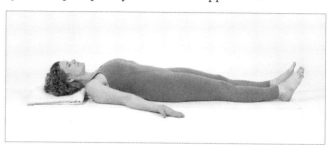

sions used for relaxation. This version uses a blanket folded in a long thin rectangle to support the torso and a second blanket to support the head.

Guided meditations that include physical relaxation are often designed to be practiced lying down. For these you can use any comfortable form of Savasana where your entire body is in contact with either the floor or with the props that are supporting you.

You can also practice any other type of meditation in a reclined position. In this case, a supported version of Savasana where your head is higher than your torso and your chest is higher than your pelvis and legs is the best position for staying alert. See Coping Skill 3: Resting Your Body and Mind with Savasana on page 28 for examples of Savasana you can use for meditation.

STANDING UP

To meditate standing up, stand in Mountain pose with your feet far enough apart—maybe hip-width apart—so your pose is as steady as possible. You can also stand with your back against a wall to increase stability. Before you begin to practice and throughout your meditation, pay attention to your posture. Maintaining the natural curves of your spine, press your feet evenly into the ground as you lengthen your spine up toward your head, and position your head directly over the top of your spine. You can keep your chest open by widening your collarbones away from each other and firming your shoulder blades against your back.

8

Making Peace with Change

When we arrive at a moment, and it is not the moment we expected, we have two options. We can accept the reality of the present moment, or we can fight it. Fighting reality leads to suffering; it's a battle we've already lost before we even start. Clinging to rigid ideas of how it was supposed to be leads to suffering. On the other hand, if we practice acceptance of reality and say, "This is not the moment I wanted, but it is the moment I am having" and we learn to be with the discomfort knowing that this moment will pass, then we suffer less. It's not that being in the present moment is always perfect—sometimes it is painful—but we can learn not to layer another level of suffering on top of the present moment by engaging in a fight against reality.

—Dr. Scott Lauzé

Taking a "yogic" approach to life means accepting the ups and downs of life with a measure of equanimity. To do this you often need to change the way you think. So many of us have been raised to believe that we can control our own destinies and that being happy means checking off bucket-list items, and we have internalized this belief. So accepting change often means adopting a different mindset.

For us in the West, yoga philosophy can provide that alternative mindset, one that we can use to make peace with change rather than "fighting with reality." Adopting a yogic understanding of human nature enables us to accept our ever-changing selves and the ever-changing world we live in. This type of acceptance does not mean resignation, however. Taking action can be the logical outcome of accepting the reality of what's happening in the present. And some of yoga's basic tenets can inspire you to engage in nonviolent social activism.

In this chapter, I'm going to offer various suggestions for ways you can change your thinking. As I mentioned in chapter 1, yoga really is much more than a set of tools. It's a system of thought—or rather a set of systems because over the thousands of years that yoga evolved it branched off in many different directions. In fact, there have been so many different paths and so many different changes to yoga over time that for us in the West things have gotten a bit confusing.

In Modern Postural Yoga (the type of yoga most of us in the West have learned), we're taught that we're following the path of Hatha Yoga, the first yoga path that emphasized the physical aspects of yoga with poses and other practices. And we're also commonly told that the yoga philosophy in Patanjali's Yoga Sutras provides the philosophical basis for practices in the Hatha Yoga path. However, Hatha Yoga originally had no relationship with the Classical Yoga of Patanjali. Instead, Hatha Yoga grew out of Tantra Yoga, which has a very different view of the universe and of what liberation means than Classical Yoga does. So I have decided to do something a bit unusual in this chapter, which is to include options from both of those traditions.

Accepting Impermanence

From the world of the senses, Arjuna, comes heat and comes cold, and pleasure and pain. They come and they go: they are transient. Arise above them, strong soul. (2.14)
—*Bhagavad Gita,* trans. Juan Mascaro

During the pandemic I realized fairly quickly that one way or another we were all facing the same dilemma: uncertainty about the future. We all had to scrap our plans and could only wait to see how things would play out. When would the pandemic end? And what would the world be like when it did?

Although I heard some people talking about various "silver linings" of the pandemic, that's not a phrase I like to use. From my point of view, there was nothing good about what was happening: people dying or suffering from long-term physical damage, people losing their jobs and their homes, and people even going hungry. And, of course, many of us were feeling scared, anxious, or angry. However, I did see a huge opportunity there, an opportunity to take to heart one of the most important lessons of yoga: that change and uncertainty are intrinsic aspects of life in the material world.

Although some were in denial and just wanted to act as if everything were still the same as it used to be, during this period most of us realized that, like it or not, the world and our lives had been forever altered. Accepting this truth that the material world is impermanent can be very hard, but it is a necessary step on the path to finding equanimity and contentment.

Refusing to accept impermanence, or "engaging in a fight against reality," as Scott Lauzé says, only increases your suffering because you will always be angry, frustrated, or depressed that things aren't the same as they once were and the future looks uncertain.

On the other hand, when you accept impermanence, yoga offers you the possibility of liberation from the suffering associated with the ever-changing material world. How you can achieve this depends on the particular yoga path that you choose to follow. But even if you decide not to go further with yoga, just accepting impermanence can allow you to navigate with greater ease through the challenges of difficult times. This has been my personal experience. As Nina Rook says:

> I don't know what the future holds for me. But I feel rooted in my community, I do the work, and I experience contentment with my life. And I experience very few nights of anxiety brought on by uncertainty about the future.
>
> The lily pad that I land on may not be the one that I had envisioned, but I know that it will have many wondrous attributes.[1]

EXPERIENCING IMPERMANENCE

Exercise: Put a drop of honey on your tongue. Notice the intensity of its flavor and observe how that flavor changes as the honey dissolves and then fades away.

In the yoga room: Traditionally Savasana, or Corpse pose, was used by yogis for contemplating impermanence and death. In modern times, because this pose typically comes as the last pose in a yoga sequence, you can use it in your own practice as a way to observe the "end" of that day's practice or to watch your breath as it arises and falls way as an embodied way to experience impermanence.

FINDING THE ETERNAL

The presence that pervades the universe
is imperishable, unchanging,
beyond both is and is not;
how could it ever vanish?

These bodies come to an end;
but that vast embodied Self
is ageless, fathomless, eternal. (2.17–18)
—*Bhagavad Gita*, trans. Stephen Mitchell

Yoga philosophy tells us that while the material world (*prakrti*) is ever changing, there is an eternal, unchanging side of the universe that you can connect with. However, in different yoga traditions, there are two very different ways of understanding the eternal, unchanging nature of the universe: dualism and nondualism.

Although it is beyond the scope of this book (and beyond my personal experience!) to provide instructions for connecting with the eternal, I thought I'd provide you with a brief overview of the two basic ways of viewing the eternal. It just makes sense to me after discussing impermanence that I should fill you in a bit on what yoga offers for those who want to follow the yoga path all the way to liberation, the very peak of the yoga mountain. I also hope this will clear up some misunderstandings about traditional yoga, which I have great respect for.

I'll start with a brief description of dualism because that is the view of the universe in Classical Yoga (the yoga described by Patanjali in the Yoga Sutras). Even though Classical Yoga wasn't originally the basis for Hatha Yoga, the yoga of Patanjali is the yoga philosophy most frequently taught these days. I'll then provide a brief description of nondualism, which actually was the basis for Hatha Yoga, as well as Tantra Yoga and Advaita Vedanta. I'll conclude with a short section about how these ideas can support you during times of change.

I'm presenting you with alternatives so you know you have a choice. But keep in mind that if you don't want to aim for a lofty spiritual goal but just want to practice yoga to make your life better here in the material world, you should feel free to do that. If you don't want to climb the whole yoga mountain, you don't have to. Just go as far as you like.

By the way, I imagine that as you read the next two sections, some of you might be wondering about the eternal in the Bhagavad Gita, a text I quote from often in this book. Is the yoga in the Gita dualism or nondualism? I wondered about that, too. Well, the answer turns out to be that we don't really know. Edwin Bryant, who is a professor of religious studies at Rutgers, says that the Gita is neither dualist nor non-dualist. The text itself doesn't even use those categories. Rather, he says, "It is the commentaries on it that are either dualist or non-dualist, and there are hundreds of commentaries on it by now from both sides of the fence."[2]

Dualism and Patanjali's Classical Yoga

In this philosophical system, everyone has their own eternal and unchanging soul, the self. While your body and mind are made from the same material as the ever-changing world around you and are therefore "painful, unclean, and temporary," your soul is immaterial and "joyful, pure, and eternal" (II.5).[3]

Although you may think of yourself as being your body and/or your mind, this is considered to be "spiritual ignorance." Your true self in this system is your "joyful, pure, and eternal" soul. And that's what you're trying to reveal by quieting your mind with your yoga practice.

According to Patanjali, you can achieve liberation from life in our ever-changing material world if you:

1. Follow the eightfold path outlined in the Yoga Sutras (or follow the alternate path of Kriya Yoga that Patanjali also describes).
2. Relinquish all your worldly attachments, including your attachments to all other people, including all family members and friends.
3. Dedicate your life to the practice of yoga.

In this path, after you move through many phases of quieting your mind, ultimately your soul will be freed from its (mistaken) association with your body-mind and will dwell for eternity in perfect aloneness (*kaivalya*), which Georg Feuerstein defines as "a trans-mental state of sheer Presence or pure Awareness."[4] Despite what you may have heard, however, this does not "unite" you with the Divine or with any other souls. If this isn't what you expected or you are disappointed by the idea of perfect aloneness, read on!

By the way, Patanjali's yoga is the most well-known dualistic yoga path, but there are others, including the Samkhya tradition and dualist Vedanta schools, which I won't be discussing in this book because they're not commonly practiced in the West.

Nondualism and Hatha Yoga, Tantra Yoga, and Advaita Vedanta

This is the state called non-dual—literally not-two—in which we can simultaneously experience the diversity of the multiverse and recognize that none of it is different from Awareness itself.

—Sally Kempton, *Meditation for the Love of It*

In this philosophical system, there is one all-encompassing universal consciousness that is eternal and unchanging, and that includes all living beings within it as well as the rest of reality. However, unlike the universal consciousness, the living beings within it, including their souls, are temporary. We are like waves in the "ocean of being," waves that arise, travel some distance, break, and then are absorbed back into the sea.

Although we live as temporary, ever-changing beings, through our practice we can experience union with the universal consciousness and the souls within it. Without dropping your body-mind or giving up your life in the material world, you can come to full realization that there is no separation between yourself, others, and the vast universal consciousness. When yoga teachers talk about how in yoga separateness is an illusion and how in reality we are all "one," this is what they are referring to.

The yoga practices of Hatha Yoga, including asanas, pranayama, meditation, and Kundalini techniques, were originally intended to allow you to experience this form of union. As Sally Kempton says:

> The ultimate effect of practice . . . is the experience of union: the union of the human consciousness with the vast Consciousness of which it is a part, or as the yogic texts put it, the recognition that there is no separation between ourselves in the whole.[5]

Coming to a temporary realization that you already are united with the universal consciousness is not something that requires arduous practice. You could experience it as you meditate and feel your boundaries dissolve or in a moment of grace. That short-lived experience may then inspire your practice. Coming to a permanent realization, which means living in our ever-changing world in a state of spiritual liberation (*jivan-mukta*), would, of course, be much harder to achieve.

By the way, there are some differences among the non-dual traditions. In Tantra, unlike Advaita Vedanta, there are three essential elements: the masculine Shiva, the passive observer of the world's movement and diversity; the feminine Shakti, the active creator of worlds, both the material and the cause; and the individual Self.

EXPERIENCING THE ETERNAL

Exercise: Resting in the pause at the end of your exhalation—the natural stage in your breath cycle when you have no more breath—is considered a way to experience the eternal. Start by observing the natural pause at the end of your exhalations and your inhalations, when you are "resting" from the actions you take while inhaling and exhaling. Then, when you feel ready, allow yourself to linger in the pause after your next exhalation. How does that stillness feel? During your rest, watch your next inhalation building and "receive" your inhalation when it feels ready. Breathe this way for a minute or more and then return to your natural breath.

Finding Comfort in the Eternal

> The little space within my heart is as great as this vast universe. The heavens and the
> earth are there, and the sun, and the moon, and the stars; fire and lightning and winds
> are there; and all that now is and all that is not: for the whole universe is in Him and He
> dwells within our heart.
>
> —Chandogya Upanishad, 8.1, trans. Juan Mascaro

Although yoga originally developed as part of Hinduism, as yoga evolved several other religions adopted yoga techniques and philosophy, including Jainism, Sikhism, and Buddhism. These days yoga is considered separate from religion and can be practiced by people of any religion or no religion at all. However, some of you may find the ideas about the eternal that I described earlier—ideas that are obviously spiritual views about the nature of the universe and human life—comforting in your everyday life.

Jivana Heyman told me that he's had moments in his practice where he feels like he has connected to something larger than his body and mind that he believes is the "eternal place" that is called the spirit. The quote above from the Chandogya Upanishad describes this essential part of him, he says, the part that hasn't changed over his entire life although his body and mind have changed—and keep changing. When he's struggling or upset, he finds it helpful to gain perspective by connecting to this place.

> It's not so much an idea, but a feeling that I reach for—the feeling of touching
> my heart. It's a similar feeling to being out in nature where I'm exposed to the
> grandeur of the sky, or the expansiveness of the stars. Getting out of my head
> is a simple way of explaining it. I remember that my perspective is so limited,
> and I have to look up from the thing I'm obsessing about to connect with the
> vastness of spirit around me, and also within me.[6]

And yoga teacher and author Barrie Risman told me that when her father died, what supported her the most was the teaching in the Bhagavad Gita and other yoga texts that in death only the physical body dies and the true Self lives on.

> The wise grieve not for those who live; and they grieve not for those who die—
> for life and earth shall pass away.

Because we all have been for all time: I, and thou, and those kings of men. And we shall be for all time, we all for ever and ever.

As the Spirit of our mortal body wanders on in childhood, and youth and old age, the Spirit wanders on to a new body: of this the sage has no doubts. (2.11–13)[7]

Barrie said that it brought her great comfort to imagine that even though her father's mortal life had ended, "his spirit was eternal and all-pervasive." She added that in some ways, "this teaching has allowed me to feel closer to him in the time since his passing than when he was alive and suffering from ill health at the end of his life."[8]

Although these are not practices that I engage in personally—and I don't think you must believe in the eternal in order to achieve equanimity and contentment—finding comfort in the eternal has been so helpful for some of my friends that I thought I'd offer these practices as possibilities for those who might be interested.

Accepting Your Thoughts and Feelings

The brain is an organ that generates thoughts and feelings all day long, one after the other, just like our hearts pump blood all day long. This process is automatic, and many of the thoughts and feelings that arise have no bearing in reality and are not "true." And yet, they feel so true because they come from deep inside of us.

—Dr. Scott Lauzé

I only recently learned about the modular view of the mind in evolutionary psychology. This theory says that because our minds gradually evolved, they developed one "module" at a time, with each module having a specialized function. With no single module in charge of the other modules, various parts of our brain are simultaneously assessing situations and reacting to them by triggering feelings and thoughts. And, at any time, a feeling or thought coming from one module might not be in agreement with feelings and thoughts coming from different modules of your brain. As Buddhists say, "thoughts think themselves."

That's why Dr. Lauzé says above that many of our thoughts and feelings have "no bearing in reality" and are not "true." Some are just reactions to a situation that triggers a response from your nervous system, such as when my cousin who lives in lower Manhattan hears helicopters circling above—a sound that she associates with 9/11—she immediately assumes something terrible must be happening. And some are thoughts triggered by your emotional state, such as when you're anxious and someone is late, and you start thinking that something terrible has surely happened to them. We may even have thoughts or feelings we don't even agree with or that make us feel ashamed, such as having fantasies about hurting other people.

Just learning to be a bit more aware of the "unreliability" of your thoughts can bring relief from suffering caused by dark thoughts. When you are troubled by worries about the future, regrets about the past, and/or judgments about the present, can you take a moment to question yourself about how true those thoughts and feelings really are? You may quickly realize that many don't reflect anything accurate about the present moment. Lately, I sometimes even find myself laughing to myself about how ridiculous some of my thoughts are, like when I found myself worrying that my mother would disapprove of my new living room furniture even though she has been dead for twelve years. We can't stop our brains from pumping out these thoughts, but we can recognize when they are stories our minds created out of our memories, fears, and hopes. My cousin, for example, understands where her panicky reactions come from—the trauma of 9/11—and that these days the sound of helicopters typically means that TV crews are covering protests in her neighborhood.

Dr. Lauzé says that it can be even more helpful if in general we can stop "overidentifying" with our minds. When you believe that all your thoughts and feelings define who you are, you create illusions about your true nature, about how much control you have over your life, and what the nature of the material world really is.

When my father was sixty three and the head of the graphic design department at a prestigious art school, he was, for political reasons, forced out of his position, a job he loved. Although he still was able to teach his classes in the department—he enjoyed teaching and working with students—a much younger and less experienced person was brought in over him. So he quit. And even though he had enough money to live on, a happy marriage, and a wonderful circle of friends, the loss of his job sent him into a depression that lasted over twenty-five years. The story he was clinging to—that he was now a failure and that his career defined who he was—prevented him from moving on and enjoying the next phase of his life.

Yoga says the same: Identifying ourselves with the thoughts and feelings we have in our minds is a false identification. This is not our true self. In Classical Yoga, ego (*asmita*) is one of the *kleshas*, the five afflictions or errors that prevent us from being able to see clearly. Barbara Stoler Miller defines *asmita* as "a false sense of self that comes about when we misidentify our essential nature with the material world."[9] Our true self in Classical Yoga is our eternal and unchanging soul, as I described earlier under Dualism and Patanjali's Classical Yoga (page 255).

In *Tantra Illuminated* Christopher Wallis says that *ahamkara*, an ancient Sanskrit term, refers to the part of the mind that identifies what is "me" and "mine." He explains that this part of our minds constructs an identity for us based on our life experiences but that "the ego is nothing more than a raft of self-images bound together by the power of your belief in them." In Tantra Yoga, you will find your true self only when you come to the realization that you are not only part of the universal consciousness but that "you are the Whole."[10]

If you're more like me and are not convinced by either of those ideas about what the true self is, you don't need to think of any part of you as being your "true self." You can simply accept yourself as a human animal who evolved to have a lot of different thoughts and feelings, some of which may be true and some of which may not be.

Whichever explanation you prefer, understanding that your thoughts and feelings don't necessarily reflect reality or define who you are can help you to better assess the real situations in front of you or within you. My student Jacqueline, whose story I'll tell in the next section, ultimately realized that the panicky thought she was having, "I'm turning into my father!" was very far from the truth, so she is now working on letting it go.

At the same time, accept that you'll always have these types of thoughts. Trying to prevent yourself from thinking certain thoughts is bound to be futile. While we can quiet our minds and shift our moods, we can't control every thought that occurs throughout our day. So don't blame yourself for continuing to have them. In *Real Change* Sharon Salzberg says these thoughts are "just visiting" and suggests you that remind yourself of this so they don't "move in."

> Once we recognize them, we can remind ourselves that they are just visiting. They are not essentially who we are. We couldn't stop them from visiting, but we can let them go. Even if they return a thousand times a session, they still have the same nature—they are visiting, we don't have to invite them to move in, we don't have to blame ourselves for their coming, and we can learn to let them go.[11]

The next section, Letting Go, provides information about how to evaluate your thoughts and feelings and the actions you can take to let them go if you determine they are not serving you.

WATCHING YOUR THOUGHTS COME AND GO

Exercise: On a partly cloudy day, take a few minutes to watch the clouds move slowly across the sky. Then, in a seated, reclined, or standing position, close your eyes and imagine the space inside your mind is a sky and that the thoughts you have are like clouds in that sky. Watch your thoughts as they form in your mind and then let them go.

In the yoga room: As you experience resistance, frustration, fear, or other challenging emotions in a yoga pose, notice those feelings and breathe through them as you stay in the pose. This is an opportunity to practice accepting your thoughts and feelings without reacting to them.

Letting Go

Abhinava Gupta argues that discernment (*tarka*) is the highest of all the limbs of yoga, and the only one that directly leads to liberation. The most important form of discernment on the spiritual path, he tells us, is discerning between what is to be held close (*upadeya*) and what is to be laid aside (*heya*)—that is, what is ultimately beneficial for you and what is not.

—Christopher Wallis, *Tantra Illuminated*

My private student Jacqueline (not her real name) confessed to me that she was feeling stuck about her online shopping "addiction," something that flared up during times of change. Even though this habit didn't cause her to overspend or cause any harm to her family, she said it still caused her great suffering. But she couldn't really explain to me what kind of suffering this habit caused her or what triggered it. I suggested that she should start by practicing some self-inquiry to learn more about what was causing the suffering and what she needed to let go of. (I'm not a therapist, but because she's a longtime yoga practitioner, we felt comfortable approaching this project in the spirit of "exploration" and "experimentation.") After that, I told her we could have some conversations about which techniques for letting go might work best for her situation and her personal preferences.

I find it fascinating that in some Tantra traditions, *tarka*, the practice of discerning between what is beneficial and what is best laid aside, is one of the six branches in the yoga path, at the same level as pranayama and meditation. Obviously this emphasis on tarka means the practice is considered essential, and it seems to me it has the potential to be very beneficial for many of us. So I've decided that even though this practice is relatively new to me, I'm going to feature it here in this chapter.

Besides "discernment," which means deciding what to lay aside, *tarka* also means "reflection" and "pondering." So it makes sense that the process of deciding what to let go of begins with self-inquiry. Before we can let go, we have to know exactly what it is we're holding on to.

I'll start this section with some suggestions for how to practice self-inquiry. I'll then present three techniques you can choose from to help you let go of what you have decided needs to be laid aside.

1. Cultivating nonattachment
2. Cultivating universal kindness
3. Cultivating forgiveness

I also want to let you know that in this section of the book I'm going to introduce some yamas you may never have heard of. As I mentioned in chapter 4, yoga teachers in the West tend to teach the five yamas listed in Patanjali's Yoga Sutras (nonviolence, truthfulness, non-stealing, non-possessiveness, and sexual restraint). However, those five yamas are not the only interesting and useful ones in the yoga tradition! Because Patanjali's five yamas have already been thoroughly covered in a wide range of modern yoga books, I decided to explore some new yamas in this chapter. I've had a wonderful time digging into them, and I hope they will inspire you.

For all the yamas—those you are familiar with and those that are new to you—I suggest you keep in mind what B. K. S. Iyengar says: "Yama is the cultivation of the positive within us."[12]

Although the yamas are called "guiding principles," it can be helpful to consider them as practices. For those yamas that speak to you, you can set an intention to begin cultivating them, both in the yoga room and in your everyday life. In this chapter, I'll provide some specific suggestions for how to practice the various yamas, but the first step, should you decide to take it, is to make practicing them your goal. As Mohandas K. Gandhi said about the yama nonviolence:

> We may never be strong enough to be entirely nonviolent in thought, word and deed. But we must keep nonviolence as our goal and make strong progress towards it.[13]

Practicing Self-Inquiry

The Witness is the lamp that illuminates all aspects of ourselves—personality and shadow, the good, the bad, the beautiful and the ugly—for understanding, acceptance, and integration. When we are able to witness our physical sensations, thoughts, emotions, and behaviors without judgment, we can cultivate and deepen our ability to recognize our patterns and consciously choose to make changes. The Witness is an integral, inseparable, indispensable part of our personal being, a true deep part of each of us that points us toward optimal health and healing

—Beth Gibbs, "Waking the Witness," *Yoga for Healthy Aging Blog*

In a self-inquiry practice, you use your witness mind, the part of your mind that allows you to impartially observe thoughts, emotions, and sensations, to study what you're experiencing. You can do this while you are practicing yoga or during a separate time you set aside to work on self-reflection. Simply focus intentionally both on what you're feeling—physically and emotionally—and on what you're thinking. Tune in to your body to observe the type of energy and the physical sensations you're experiencing. Allow yourself to fully experience your emotions and observe the thoughts those emotions trigger.

During this process, try to employ radical honesty, observing what you feel and think without shame or any kind of judgment. In the Yoga Yajnavalkya, Hatha Yoga Pradipika, and other yoga texts, one of the ten yamas is *arjava* (honesty), and practicing this type of honesty can be a good way to really get to the bottom of things.

If you're familiar with Patanjali's five yamas, you might be wondering what the difference is between the "honesty" that is arjava and the "truthfulness" that is the satya (one of Patanjali's five yamas). There is a meaningful difference. While *satya* means speaking the factual truth when communicating with others and not engaging in lying, *arjava* means being honest with yourself and respecting what you know to be true for you at this moment in time. Christopher Wallis described it this way:

> I wouldn't really know why I was depressed until I did self-enquiry, a self-enquiry whose ability to pierce through to reality was greatly aided by radical honesty—the kind of honesty that comes only when I drop any sense of shame to be thinking anything so absurd as what I had been thinking.[14]

As I mentioned in chapter 4, in a Tantra Yoga tradition, all thoughts and feelings are considered opportunities for learning about yourself. Taking that approach may allow you to let go of any shame you feel about having thoughts or emotions that you consider "negative."

When you've finished with this process of witnessing without judgment, you can step back and use your wisdom mind (*buddhi*) to discern what you need to let go of. Your buddhi is the analytical part of your mind—your intellect—that you use to reason, discern, and judge. In the yoga tradition, the buddhi is not located only in your brain, but is distributed throughout your body. I like this idea because it means you can use "gut feelings" to make your decisions. Maybe you'll know right away what needs letting go! Or maybe you'll have to "let it sit and simmer," as Beth Gibbs says, until you reach clarity.

The following two sections provide further suggestions about when and how to practice self-inquiry.

WHEN TO PRACTICE SELF-INQUIRY

No matter who we are, where we live, or what our current condition or situation is, our ability to witness what is happening in the moment enables us to respond appropriately to the ups and downs of our human experience in a wise and balanced manner. This is true whether it's a situation with our physical body, our energy, or our mind and emotions.

—Beth Gibbs, "Waking the Witness," *Yoga for Healthy Aging Blog*

A dedicated self-inquiry session can be any amount of quiet time you set aside to work on self-reflection, either during your yoga practice or at another time. In your yoga practice, you can practice self-inquiry by "sitting" with your thoughts and feelings in meditation or observing them while you are practicing yoga poses. (I have learned a lot about my feelings of fear in my yoga practice by intentionally practicing poses that scared me and watching the same feelings come up over and over.)

Barrie Risman says that *after* she practices her yoga poses she finds it helpful to take a minute or two to "become aware of and articulate the effects of the practice." She will try to notice and describe how she feels after the practice, how the practice affected her, and whether she shifted in any way, whether physically, mentally, or emotionally. She will either write down her observations or just silently articulate them to herself. She says this practice helps "clarify the beneficial effects and strengthens commitment."[15]

Separate from your yoga practice, you can practice self-inquiry by:

- Writing in a journal.
- Drawing, painting, or using any creative project to explore your thoughts and feelings.
- Taking a walk and allowing yourself to explore your thoughts and feelings in a relaxed and unstructured way.
- Talking through some issues with the right friend. (I haven't seen this idea mentioned elsewhere, but I think talking through your concerns with a trusted friend who can listen without judgment could help you discover what you need to let go of.)

Dr. Scott Lauzé says that practicing self-inquiry in any of these ways can enable you to become an "expert" on yourself and to learn to respond more skillfully to your thoughts and emotions, rather than just automatically reacting:

Meditation, mindful movement, journaling, creative projects are all practices that help us to be present and observe what arises in our thinking and in our bodies. We become our own psychiatrists, experts on our own minds. We get some distance from our thoughts, develop a healthy skepticism, and learn which thoughts lead to suffering. We become less reactive, more thoughtful.[16]

For her self-inquiry regarding what was causing her suffering, Jacqueline ended up using several of the techniques I suggested here, including meditating, writing in a journal, talking with a trusted friend, and thinking while she took walks. She eventually realized that stress triggered her to buy things she felt she didn't actually "need." For example, at the beginning of the pandemic, she ordered several of her favorite shoes as well as some extra clothes "just in case." So, as the pandemic continued, she began to practice Legs Up the Wall pose at the end of every day as a healthier coping strategy for stress.

But she also realized that the actual "suffering" occurred when what she ordered arrived at her house and she would panic, thinking "I'm turning into my father!" Her father, she explained to me, had suffered from lifelong depression and had also been a serious hoarder, filling up their house and multiple cars with his stuff, which as a child made her ashamed to have anyone over. And even though Jacqueline never had mental health problems and wasn't a hoarder—she had a happy, busy life and beautiful, well-organized home—having packages arrive at her house triggered shame, guilt, and panic. And really, even when she was trying to follow a strict "no-buy" policy, it never seemed possible to reduce her shopping to a level that felt comfortable to her. So, there was also some "baggage" she needed to let go of.

HOW TO PRACTICE SELF-INQUIRY

When you're suffering or feeling "uncomfortable," you can focus your self-inquiry on your situation to find out more about what's going on with you and see if you can identify what is not serving you. You may be currently experiencing that suffering or discomfort, in which case you can simply observe yourself in the present. But if you're not currently having the experience, you can consciously allow yourself to go back to a time when you were.

There's no formula for this self-inquiry process that I know of, so you can feel free just to do what feels right to you. But if you can't figure out what to do or just want some fresh ideas, here are some basic questions to explore. You can use these suggestions in your yoga practice or while meditating, or in a separate self-reflection session when you write in a journal, do a creative project, take a walk, or just sit with your thoughts.

Caution: Dr. Scott Lauzé says that these practices are not right for everyone, warning that "People who struggle with psychotic illnesses, or who have suffered from trauma that has not been processed in therapy, may not benefit from this kind of deep inward-looking and should consult with professionals before proceeding."[17]

What Is Your Body Telling You?

Your physical responses to situations that are challenging can provide you with quite a bit of information. Try observing your energy levels, your breath, and your physical symptoms, if any.

Energy. A good place to start is with your energy levels. At the beginning of the pandemic, I was so exhausted all the time, even though I felt I was very lucky in my situation compared to so many other people in the world (we could work at home, had enough money, had enough space, and so on.). Eventually I realized that the gratitude practices I'd been employing to get through the stress of sheltering in place meant that I'd been stuffing down my feelings of anxiety, stress, concern for others, and other painful feelings. It was only when I reached this understanding and admitted how I was feeling that I was able to address the reality of my situation.

Breath. Observing your breath provides you with information about your emotional state. Are you breathing slowly or rapidly? Is your breath smooth and even or is it jagged and rough?

Physical symptoms. For many of us, stress and emotional distress causes physical symptoms. In chapter 4, Jivana Heyman described typical physical symptoms of anxiety, including headaches and digestive problems. And a big warning sign for me is a burning sensation I get in my chest when I'm very stressed out; I know this is my body's way of telling me it's time to double down on relaxation practices. Of course, you can't always correlate your physical symptoms with an emotional state—sometimes you might just be ill, for example—but observing them over time may help you make some useful connections.

What Are Your Emotions Telling You?

We tend to fill our minds with fear, worry, anxiety, grief, anger, rage, jealousy, and judgments, among others, and we do not let go of these emotions. Over time, these emotions—whether they are bitterness, fear, emotional damage, rejection or abandonment—build up. If you hoard/accumulate unexpressed or suppressed emotions and if they are not getting released, they keep building up in your body.

—Dr. Ram Rao, "Aparigraha (Non-Hoarding) and Healthy Aging,"
Yoga for Healthy Aging Blog

Although most emotions are very strong, I think our feelings of shame about having certain "negative" emotions can prevent us from acknowledging them. I remember that even though my husband was immediately angry with my father about how he behaved toward my mother while she was dying, it took me a long time to admit to myself that I was feeling the same way. But obviously you can't let go of an emotion if you don't first acknowledge that you're experiencing it. So, practicing arjava—honesty with yourself—is especially valuable when observing your emotions. And I think it can be helpful to think of these types of emotions as "painful" rather than "negative" and to remind yourself that in some yoga traditions all feelings are considered opportunities for learning about ourselves.

Remember how in chapter 1 I described how we evolved to experience attraction to and aversion for everything and everyone in our environment, and also how compelling our urge to plan for the future is? All these primal impulses cause strong emotions. So try to see how the emotions you're experiencing relate to basic aversion, attraction, and planning for the future because that may give you hints about what you need to let go of.

What Are Your Thoughts Telling You?

The things in your environment—the sights, the sounds, the smells, the people, the news, the videos—are pushing your buttons, activating feelings that, however subtly, set in motion trains of thought and reaction that govern your behavior, sometimes in ways that are unfortunate. And they will keep doing that unless you start paying attention to what's going on.

—Robert Wright, *Why Buddhism Is True*

As described in chapter 3, your primal impulses and reactions to stress have very strong effects on your thoughts. So observing your thought patterns—and noticing the origins of those thoughts—can be very helpful for identifying what you need to let go of.

Because shame can sometimes cause problems with your ability to acknowledge what you're really thinking, practicing the yama arjava—honesty with yourself—is also especially valuable when you are observing your thoughts. See if you can find patterns: Are you mostly thinking about the past? If so, with nostalgia or regrets? Are you mostly thinking about the future? If so, with anxiety or by having pleasurable fantasies? Or are you in the present but constantly making instantaneous judgments about what's "good" or "bad"? You can then consider which of the thoughts you're having are helpful and which are not.

Through her process, Jacqueline ultimately realized that the thought "I'm turning into my father" she kept having was both untrue and not helpful. She was, in fact, nothing like her father, and occasionally buying something she didn't "need" wasn't harming either herself or her family. But the difficulties of her childhood in Canada, which included living with a mentally ill parent who sometimes scared her, had left her with fears that kept triggering this thought. She realized now that it was time to let that thought go.

Of course, practicing this type of self-exploration may not be the best way or only way for you to find the answers you're looking for. So if you ultimately realize that you need professional help, don't hesitate to seek it out. You may even be able to combine self-inquiry with therapy.

CULTIVATING NONATTACHMENT (*VAIRAGYA*)

Vairagya is a way of putting the gears of the mind into neutral, disengaging ourselves from the thoughts, feelings, and desires that normally hook our attention.

—Sally Kempton, *Meditation for the Love of It*

At the very end of the movie *The Darjeeling Limited*, the three brothers who are traveling through India and who have been grieving the death of their father for a very long time, are running to catch a train. The luggage they are carrying as they run—which is marked with their father's initials and some of which contains his personal items—is slowing them down, so eventually all three just toss the baggage aside. They are then able to reach the train and jump on board. In a way, it's that simple to let go of thoughts and emotions that you realize aren't serving you.

Jacqueline, who realized she was being tormented by the untrue thought—triggered by bad memories of her childhood—that she was turning into her father, who was a hoarder and had mental illness problems, came up with the idea of letting go of that thought by picturing this very movie scene, which she watched on YouTube. She says:

> For me, I visualize the smirk on the brother's face when the other brother tells him they need to toss the luggage to make the train. It is like, oh yeah, I get to dump this crap and be happy about it!

The term *vairagya*, which means renunciation as well as nonattachment, is one of the yamas in the Trishikhi Brahmana Upanishad. To practice this yama, there are a number of specific techniques that you can try.

If you meditate regularly, the practice of concentration teaches you to notice your thoughts and emotions and then let them go by returning your focus to your object of meditation. So in your meditation practice you can intentionally work with releasing unhelpful thoughts and emotions. At the beginning of your session, you can set an intention to let go of all thoughts and emotions, and then practice this repeatedly throughout your meditation. From this practice, you may learn how you can just "disengage" from your thoughts and emotions in everyday life in the same way. You can use many different meditation techniques to do this, including any of the techniques I'm suggesting here in this section or techniques you learn from a teacher.

If you don't have a regular meditation practice, you can still choose from any of the following techniques to practice letting go throughout your day. Like any other skill, the more you practice letting go, the better you'll get at it. For more than twenty-five years, I've been telling myself "Don't panic too soon" when I notice myself getting swept away by anxious thoughts about the future. It still makes me laugh a little and sets me back on track.

Here are some techniques for letting go:

1. **Use your breath.** You can use your breath at any time to release an unhelpful thought or emotion with your exhalation. Simply inhale and then, with your exhalation, breathe out that thought or emotion. If needed, you can repeat the process with more breaths.

2. **Picture an action.** You can use a mental image that says "let go" to release unhelpful thoughts and emotions. Some ideas include moving your thought or emotion into

a trash can like you do on your computer or putting it on a log and watching it float down a river. You can even get creative and use a scene like the one from *The Darjeeling Limited*, that says "letting go of baggage" to you. Barrie Risman says that she likes to visualize "offering" unhelpful thoughts and emotions to a fire.

3. **Recite a phrase.** You can select any quote from a yoga text or a quote from somewhere else to recite mentally. Or you can make something up yourself, the way I did with "Don't panic too soon."

4. **Tune in to your senses.** One way to let go of thoughts or emotions regarding the past or future is to bring yourself into the present by immersing yourself in a sensory experience, such as exploring all aspects of a flower, a cup of tea, a peach, or a book (did you ever smell a book?).

5. **Cultivate the opposite.** Sutra II.33 in Patanjali's Yoga Sutras recommends the practice of *pratipaksha bhavana*, which means "cultivate the opposite" or "cultivate counteracting thoughts," as a way to let go of negative thoughts and emotions. With this practice, you intentionally think an opposite thought, one that is more helpful than the original thought or emotion. For example, maybe you find yourself thinking "I can't deal with this!" You could intentionally follow that with a thought like "I can be okay with this." This practice has long-term benefits because you spend more time thinking positive thoughts and feeling positive emotions, which can start a new habit for you. If you have problems with coming up with "opposite" thoughts, read the next two sections for ideas.

6. **In the yoga room.** You can practice letting go when you practice yoga poses by bringing your awareness to the endings of poses. When you come out of a pose, consciously release the thoughts, feelings, and experiences you had while practicing the pose as well as judgments about your performance. Come back to the present moment before moving to the next pose.

CULTIVATING UNIVERSAL KINDNESS

By cultivating an attitude of friendship toward those who are happy, compassion toward those in distress, joy toward those who are virtuous, and equanimity toward those who are nonvirtuous, lucidity arises in the mind. (I.33)

—Edwin Bryant, *The Yoga Sutras of Patanjali*

As we experience change—or simply move from one stage of life to another—what often interferes with our ability to be content are the feelings we have when we compare ourselves to others. If we're honest with ourselves, we'll admit that comparing ourselves to others can lead to some ugly feelings, including envy, jealousy, anger, and intolerance. Sometimes we even have violent thoughts or feelings of ill will. Ancient yogis recognized this. According to Edwin Bryant,

> Hariharananda suggests that envy generally arises when we encounter people whom we do not care about experiencing happiness. Even a pious person can invoke our jealousy and we take cruel delight when we find an enemy in misery.[18]

But according to Patanjali by cultivating positive feelings for those who trigger the negative ones, we can "remove" the negative feelings that are disturbing our equanimity. Sutra I.33, quoted above, says that the reason for conducting yourself with friendship, compassion, sympathetic joy, and equanimity toward others is to allow "lucidity" to arise in your mind (not just to be a good person). And Edwin Bryant describes practicing this sutra as an "off-the-mat type of meditation" for quieting the mind.

Yes, these four practices are the same as the Buddhist four *brahmavihara*, the divine abodes that are sometimes called the four aspects of love. These four practices, which you can think of as yamas, allow you to train your heart. Your ability to feel friendship (also known as loving-kindness), compassion, sympathetic joy, and equanimity increases with practice and even changes the structure of your brain. In *The Wisdom of Yoga*, Stephen Cope describes it this way:

> The more we practice loving kindness, compassion, sympathetic joy, happiness, the stronger they become. The part of the brain that supports these states is strengthened and becomes more robust. As these wholesome states are being practiced, the difficult negative states, involving quite a different set of neural connections, are waning in strength, dominance, and physical development.[19]

Cultivating these states might improve your relationships, as you can become kinder and less reactive. And they may also inspire you to take action in the world, turning unconditional friendship and compassion for others into force for change. See The Path of Karma Yoga on page 255 for more information.

The following sections discuss each of the four practices individually. See Cultivating Forgiveness on page 252 for a fifth practice that you might also find helpful.

Cultivating Unconditional Friendship (*Maitri*)

In daily life we see people around who are happier than we are, people who are less happy.... Whatever may be our usual attitude toward such people and their actions, if we can be pleased with others who are happier than ourselves . . . our mind will be very tranquil. (I.33)

—Patanjali, trans. T. K. V. Desikachar, *The Heart of Yoga*

When you experience loss, it can be hard to witness the happiness of others, especially those who have what you once had or who have what you've always wanted. You might feel envy—a very painful emotion—or even secretly wish some harm would befall the people you envy.

For your peace of mind, sutra I.33 tells you instead to cultivate *maitri* for those who are happy. While Edwin Bryant translates *maitri* in sutra I.33 as "friendship," another translation is "loving-kindness." This is the benevolent desire for well-being and happiness for others as well as for yourself. This practice complements ahimsa, nonviolence. In addition to just refraining from thoughts of harming others, you should wish them well.

As one of the four virtues of Buddhism, loving-kindness, known as *metta* as well as maitri, is often cultivated on behalf of all beings. As a yoga practitioner, you should feel free to practice this way, too. However, in the context of yoga sutra I.33, this practice is about letting go of negative thoughts and emotions regarding those who are happy (or happier than you).

Cultivating this same unconditional friendship for yourself can not only help you let go of negative thoughts and emotions you have for yourself but can also train you to extend that feeling to others. According to Pema Chödrön,

It is never too late or too early to practice loving-kindness. It is said that we can't attain enlightenment, let alone feel contentment and joy, without seeing who we are and what we do, without seeing our patterns and our habits. This is called maitri—developing loving-kindness and an unconditional friendship with ourselves.[20]

Here are some ways you might practice unconditional friendship:

1. **Cultivating the opposite.** You can use thoughts of loving-kindness as your "opposite thoughts" as described under Cultivating Nonattachment on page 242.
2. **Acts of friendship.** Through acts of unconditional friendship, small and large, you can support the happiness of others.
3. **Loving-kindness meditation.** You can use a guided loving-kindness meditation that you find in a book or recording. Or you can choose your own phrases of loving-kindness in your meditation as you picture first yourself, someone you love, a neutral person, and finally a difficult person.
4. **In the yoga room.** To cultivate unconditional friendship toward yourself, you can just take a moment, either at the beginning or end of practice, or even after every pose, to thank yourself for showing up.

Jacqueline, whose suffering over her online shopping I described earlier, realized during her self-inquiry she was very hard on herself for "slipping up" whenever she bought anything that she considered strictly unnecessary. So she decided to practice her own, customized version of the loving-kindness meditation to cultivate kindness toward herself. As she thought of living with ease, she imagined letting go of the burden of thinking she was like her father. And she added this phrase to the meditation: "May I be kind to myself and others."

Cultivating Compassion (*Karuna*)

Compassion for the suffering of others is more than just sympathy. . . . Real compassion is potent as it implies the question, "What can I do to help?"

—B. K. S. Iyengar, *Light on Life*

To let go of the negative emotions you feel toward those in distress, sutra I.33 recommends practicing compassion (*karuna*). Unlike simple pity or concern, feeling compassion means experiencing the sufferings of others as if they were your own. This can help you improve your relationships with those in distress as well as those with whom you have difficult relationships because compassion allows you to understand the fears and desires that are motivating others.

(You might wonder, who ever has negative feelings about people who are suffering? Well, I confess to having angry feelings about unhoused people who leave huge piles of garbage around our city, which I try to counteract with compassion.)

And having compassion for yourself allows you to let go of guilt about mistakes you've made and shame about feelings you think you should not be having. As Dr. Lauzé says:

> We are human, we take wrong turns sometimes, but it's the wrong turns that teach us how to move forward more skillfully. Self-compassion about our imperfections, and compassion about the imperfections of others, brings relief.[21]

Unlike the word *compassion* in English, which just means experiencing the suffering of others as your own, the word *karuna* in Sanskrit includes taking action to alleviate that suffering. In fact, the idea of taking action based on compassionate feelings is built into the word *karuna*. According to Pandit Rajmani Tigunait, *karu* means "action, endeavor, ability to do" and *na* means "to move forward, to lead, leading capacity, the process of reaching a destination."

> Together *karuna* refers to an action or virtue that enables you to move forward; the virtue that compels you to help others move forward; the virtue that compels you to pull others out of their misery; the virtue that compels you to extend yourself to those who are stuck; compassion.[22]

So practicing compassion not only means cultivating compassionate feelings for others, but also taking actions to relieve their suffering. This is a completely selfless form of compassionate action, from which you do not expect anything in return, not even gratitude. Charissa Loftis says that she was finally able to let go of her anger at her father, a Vietnam War veteran, by cultivating compassion for him and taking action to relieve his suffering by giving him yoga therapy for his COPD.

Here are some ways you might practice compassion:

1. **Cultivating the opposite.** You can use compassionate thoughts as your "opposite thoughts" as described under Cultivating Nonattachment on page 242.
2. **Helping others.** Take any appropriate actions to help individuals who are suffering or organizations that support them. Offer your emotional support, your time, your skills, your money, or anything else that might help. To practice this compassion in action the yogic way, keep the principles of Karma Yoga in mind (see The Path of Karma Yoga on page 255).
3. **Compassion meditation.** In a compassion meditation, you focus on a person or a group of people who are suffering or experiencing difficulty, and then wish for a positive outcome for them. You can make up your own or look for a formal compassion meditation. Of course, because you can't help everyone in the world for whom you feel compassion, cultivating compassion for yourself about that could also be helpful.
4. **In the yoga room.** When you practice yoga poses, you can consciously cultivate compassion for yourself. At the beginning of your practice, as you are rolling out your mat, clearing your space, or taking your first pose, welcome yourself to your practice with compassion for how you are feeling in the moment. And as you practice your poses, give yourself permission to make a pose easier or more accessible by using props to support yourself or by choosing a variation that feels better for you at the current time.

Cultivating Sympathetic Joy (*Mudita*)

Just as we may feel envy for those who are happier than we are, we can feel the same for those who are more accomplished or those who, as Desikachar says, are doing "praiseworthy" things. Sutra I.33 tells us to cultivate joy instead for those who are virtuous. Although *mudita* is often translated simply as "joy" or "happiness," it is actually the special kind of unselfish joy that you feel when you are happy for someone else, even when you played no part in that person's accomplishments and they won't benefit you personally. The example that is most often used to illustrate sympathetic joy is the joy a parent feels when their child accomplishes something significant, gets a lucky break, or finds happiness.

Practicing sympathetic joy for family members may be easy, but practicing it outside of your inner circle can be challenging. Probably because of primal urges dating back to when we were competing over scarce resources, we often experience the success and happiness of those we see as "rivals" as threatening. This can cause envy and even ill wishes for those you are envious of (and then the shame that comes with having ill wishes). But rising to this challenge and cultivating sympathetic joy can help you let go of negative emotions you feel when good things happen to other people.

This reminds me of a story Jivana Heyman tells about how his original motivation for creating the Accessible Yoga community was envy. When he moved to Santa Barbara, California, and had to start up his yoga teaching career again from scratch, he felt envious of the other yoga teachers who had successful careers teaching what he himself wanted to teach. So, inspired by pratipaksha bhavana, the yogic practice of cultivating the opposite, what he decided to do was to create a venue where these very teachers—the ones he envied—could do their good work.

Here are some ways you might practice sympathetic joy:

1. Cultivating the opposite. You can use thoughts of sympathetic joy as your "opposite thoughts" as described under Cultivating Nonattachment on page 242.
2. Celebrating others. Engage in actions that support and celebrate the achievements of others.
3. Mudita meditation. In a mudita meditation, you mentally recite phrases of sympathetic joy, such as "I'm happy for you" and "May your happiness continue," as you picture first someone you love, then a person for whom you have neutral feelings, and finally a difficult person. If you're interested, you can look for a formal mudita meditation.

Cultivating Equanimity (*Upeksanam* or *Upeksa*)

Whatever may be our usual attitude toward such people and their actions, if we can be pleased with others who are happier than ourselves, compassionate toward those who are unhappy, joyful with those doing praiseworthy things, and remain undisturbed by the errors of others, our mind will be very tranquil. (I.33)

—Patanjali, trans. T. K. V. Desikachar, *The Heart of Yoga*

Sutra I.33 addresses your relationship with "non-virtuous" people by saying that we should cultivate equanimity toward them. The "equanimity" this sutra refers to is the same as the "evenness of mind" that the Bhagavad Gita recommends for facing life's ups and downs.

If you're wondering who the non-virtuous might be, consider that the five basic yamas in the Yoga Sutras (nonviolence, truthfulness, non-stealing, non-possessiveness, and sexual continence) define the "virtuous." Therefore, the non-virtuous would include anyone who intentionally harms others, whether through violence, lies, greed, theft, or sexual abuse.

To let go of the negative emotions you feel toward these people, you don't need to cultivate unconditional friendship or compassion; instead, just work on disengaging from the anger, hatred, and other unpleasant emotions you might be feeling for them. As a longtime practitioner of yoga and nonviolence, Mohandas K. Gandhi was committed to non-hatred of the British people, whose government had oppressed the people of India for so many years. In his "Quit India" speech, he said, "Our quarrel is not with the British people, we fight their imperialism," and "Speaking for myself, I can say that I have never felt any hatred."[23]

Taking a more "neutral" stance not only can allow you to stay balanced and steady yourself, but can also enable you to observe the non-virtuous with clearer eyes. If appropriate, you can then take action to stop them from causing harm to you or to others. This, of course, is what Gandhi did to win India's independence from British colonial rule.

Here are some ways you might cultivate this neutral stance:

1. **Letting go.** To let go of hatred, anger, and other negative emotions you feel toward the non-virtuous, you can use any appropriate techniques described for Cultivating Nonattachment (page 242).
2. **Forgiveness.** For those who have hurt you or others you care about, you can cultivate kshama, yoga's yama of forgiveness, a form of letting go that I will describe next.
3. **Concentration meditation.** You can cultivate more evenness of mind by meditating with a focus on peace, for example, by using the mantra OM SHANTI or SHANTI, SHANTI, SHANTI. And during this practice, if negative feelings arise, you can let them go as you return your focus to meditating on peace.

4. Mindfulness meditation. Teachers of mindfulness meditation say that you can dissipate some negative feelings if you focus on them during your practice. The simple act of paying close attention to them can reduce their power.

Cultivating Forgiveness (*Kshama*)

Once we realize that by inwardly blessing an enemy we can melt our own anger and resentment, we no longer feel like such victims of our feelings.
—Sally Kempton, *Meditation for the Love of It*

When there is someone who caused you or people you care about to lose something important—whether that's a marriage or other relationship, a job or a home, feelings of self-confidence, or the ability to feel safe—it can be hard to let go completely of your anger or resentment at the person who caused the harm. You may be reminded over and over of the crime committed against you or those you care about or of how someone betrayed you.

This happened to Ram Rao and his wife Padma. After experiencing some traumatic events, they suffered from ongoing reminders that included intense memories and even flashbacks of the "harrowing" experiences. In an attempt to "overlay" their painful memories with positive feelings and experiences, they practiced yoga, meditation, pranayama, Ayurveda, and pranic healing. Although this brought them closer to alleviating the traumatic experiences, Ram said, "At the very far corner of our minds, we continued to harbor the negativity, albeit at a low threshold."

It was only when Ram and Padma learned about kshama (forgiveness) and began to put this yama into practice that they were able to finally let go completely of the traumatic experiences and move on. Now Ram says:

Over the years, forgiving actually helped us to erase that little speck of negativity that was deeply rooted in the far corner of our brains and brought us to a more 'present state.' We could completely mitigate our past horrible experiences through the act of forgiveness, and gone was the sorrow, sadness, and flashbacks. The harrowing events disappeared completely; it was as if the nerves associated with these experiences had either withdrawn completely or had died down.

We understood that since the biggest obstacle to connecting with our true selves was hatred or bitterness, forgiving the individuals who injured our minds and upset our emotional balance helped us to let go of the underlying emotions. Let me clarify that by forgiving, we were neither accepting nor forgetting the facts. Forgiveness also doesn't mean we were overlooking/excusing the behavior or that we were correcting the wrong. Forgiveness only meant that we needed to free ourselves from the traumatic past and move on with those events cleared from our lives.[24]

Kshama is one of the ten yamas in the Yoga Yajnavalkya, the Hatha Yoga Pradipika, and other yoga texts. The Sanskrit word *kshama* is especially beautiful because it has so many layers of meaning. In addition to being "forgiveness," it also means "letting go, releasing time, and living in the present." As you can see from Ram's story, by forgiving those who have harmed you or others, you are able to let go of your attachment to a grievance and release the grip the past has on you. The word also means "forbearance," no doubt because the ability to forgive and let go allows you to bear so much more with patience and large-heartedness.

Practicing kshama does not mean confronting or reconciling with the person or people who caused harm. Instead, it is a type of forgiveness that you practice within yourself so you can "release" the pain associated with the harm that was done to you or to others you care about, and then to move on from it. Of course, if you have harmed yourself or done something that you regret, you can also forgive yourself.

Here are three ways you might practice kshama:

1. Meditation. You can use a loving-kindness meditation and focus on the person who caused harm when you reach that point in the meditation. You could also just focus solely on the person who caused you harm (or on yourself) in your meditation, using any phrase you feel best expresses your forgiveness and a letting go of the hurt they caused (or that you caused).

2. Cultivating the opposite. Each time you notice yourself remembering how someone harmed you, you could intentionally follow that thought with an "opposite" thought, such as "I forgive that person," "I'm releasing this now," or whatever phrase works for you. You can do the same for yourself if it is yourself you need to forgive.

3. Acts of charity. You could take charitable actions in your life, such as making donations or doing a charitable deed, in honor of the person whom you want to forgive.

Taking Action

Arriving at a moment and accepting it as it is doesn't mean that we become spineless jellyfish or doormats. If some injustice is happening, or we are experiencing suffering that is in our power to change, then we absolutely can take action in the present moment to get us closer to our goals moving forward.

—Dr. Scott Lauzé

After coming down with type 1 diabetes at the age of thirty-five, Melitta Rorty decided to take two types of actions:

1. She would do the best possible job of taking care of her health, including eating the best foods, exercising regularly, and carefully managing her blood sugar levels via blood tests and insulin injections.
2. Because she had initially been misdiagnosed as having type 2 diabetes, which does not require insulin, and had almost died as a result, she vowed to increase public awareness that type 1 diabetes can occur in adults of any age as well as in children and to advocate for changes in the medical establishment in the way adults with type 1 are diagnosed and treated.

So the major change in her health status prompted Melitta to take both personal actions and engage in social activism.

As I said at the beginning of this chapter, accepting change doesn't mean refraining from taking action. In fact, because just living in the world (even in a cave) means taking actions, day in and day out, there is no way to escape the need to act. In the Bhagavad Gita, Krishna explains that this is the nature of life in the material world:

No one, not even for an instant,
can exist without acting: all beings
are compelled, however unwilling,
by the three strands of Nature called *gunas*. (3.5)[25]

So, to allow you to maintain peace of mind—even as you work to make changes in your own life and/or in the world—there is a yogic approach to taking action: choosing the "right" actions and practicing Karma Yoga, the yoga of action, when you do act.

Choosing the "right" actions is something you each have to work through on your own. However, you can use the yamas, yoga's ethical guidelines, to help make decisions. Considering the five yamas in the Yoga Sutras (nonviolence, truthfulness, non-stealing, non-possessiveness, and sexual responsibility), the additional yamas I've discussed in this book—and any others you learn about—can guide you in doing what's right for yourself, your family, your community, and the world.

As for practicing the yoga of action, Karma Yoga, this is the main subject of one of the most important yoga texts of them all, the Bhagavad Gita.

THE PATH OF KARMA YOGA

In this world there are two main paths:
the yoga of understanding,
for contemplative men; and for men
who are active, the yoga of action. (3.3)
—*Bhagavad Gita,* trans. Stephen Mitchell

Although in the West we commonly hear that the eightfold path outlined in the Yoga Sutras is the yoga path we should all be following, this is not the only yoga path, and it might not be the right one for you. I'm not saying that wisdom of the Yoga Sutras has no value for us—I think it certainly does—but I've concluded that the eightfold path is not one that we householders can follow in a literal way. First of all, we would have to become renunciants because even being attached to people you love, including your family, interferes with your ability to achieve liberation. And the path—with its intended goal of liberation from everyday life as we know it—is really quite arduous and severe because we would eventually have to let go of all connection to external reality.

On the other hand, the Bhagavad Gita describes a different path, the path of Karma Yoga, which seems more suitable for householders (*grihastha-yogin*), people with livelihoods, families, and communities who have important work to do in the world. (It's called Karma Yoga, by the way, because *karma* literally means "action" in Sanskrit.)

Arjuna, the focus of the Bhagavad Gita and the person to whom the god-man Krishna reveals the wisdom of yoga, is himself very much a householder. He is married to several women and has children and a large extended family he cares about. His profession is that of a warrior (he is the son of Indra, the great warrior deity), and he has fought many battles in the past. And the battle that he is about to enter at the start of the Bhagavad Gita is a war that Arjuna believes in; he is fighting for his family to win back the kingdom that was stolen from them so that his brother Yudhishthira can take his rightful place on the throne. So Arjuna is very much engaged with the world, and he is facing a dilemma that is metaphorical for the situations all of us face at one time or another.

Although Arjuna is poised to fight an actual war, you can think of the impending battle in the Gita as any kind of situation you find yourself in that compels you to take action. For example, Melitta Rorty took on two different battles: the challenges of self-care required by having type 1 diabetes and her goal of eliminating misdiagnosis of adult-onset type 1 diabetes by the medical establishment.

Even though Arjuna is fighting for what he believes is a righteous cause, he pauses in despair before entering the fight, afraid of the collateral damage he might cause—the possible death of relatives and beloved teachers he sees on the opposite side. When he confesses this to his friend, Krishna urges Arjuna not to withdraw from the battle but to enter into it as part of his yogic path. And he then advises Arjuna how to fight for what he believes is right with equanimity rather than being tormented by his fears for what the results of his actions might be. Krishna says to him:

> The wise man lets go of all
> results, whether good or bad,
> and is focused on the action alone.
> Yoga is skill in actions. (2.50)

Practicing skill in action means focusing solely on the action you're taking, without worrying about what the end results will be. It also means accepting the results of your action, whether success or failure, with equanimity.

> Self-possessed, resolute, act
> without any thoughts of results,

open to success or failure.
This equanimity is yoga. (2.48)[26]

Krishna goes on to say that Arjuna should take this yogic approach for all the actions he takes in his life. You, too, can adopt this philosophy to help you stay calm and steady as you take whatever actions you choose to take—or need to take—in life. These can be any actions: small or large, personal or on behalf of others. In some cases, this philosophy may give you the courage to stand up for what's right, as it did for Arjuna and, at other times, you may simply be transforming your everyday life. As Georg Feuerstein says:

> If we apply ourselves to the principles of Karma-Yoga, we may well find, as Sri Aurobindo noted, that our actions remain outwardly the same. The real work we are challenged to undertake concerns our inner life. Yet, our new disposition will inevitably shine through our actions as well. We may still perform the same steps in washing dishes, for instance, but our movements and comportment will be calm and balanced.[27]

By the way, the quote that opens this section mentions only two yoga paths, but there are actually many others these days—in fact, too many to list.

THE ROYAL ROAD: SERVICE AND SOCIAL JUSTICE

In discussing compassion earlier in this chapter, I said that in the yoga tradition compassion not only means feeling the suffering of others as your own, but it also includes taking action to alleviate that suffering. This is why acts of service for others and working for social justice are an integral part of yoga. Here's how Mohandas K. Gandhi put it:

> It is man's nature to do good, for all selves are one. Man's essence, which is Atman, is all-pervading. He who has realized this will not see himself as different from others, but will see all in himself. For such a person, therefore, doing good becomes his nature.[28]

Of course, Gandhi himself is known worldwide for his work as a social activist and for developing the practice of nonviolent passive resistance (*satyagraha*), which inspired the social activism of Martin Luther King Jr. and Nelson Mandela, among others. What is not as widely known is that his lifelong work as a social activist was inspired by his practice of Karma Yoga as described in the Bhagavad Gita.

This meant that in all the social activism in which Gandhi engaged, whether he was fighting for the independence of India or working for religious harmony in the country after independence was achieved, he practiced skill in action. He aimed to do his work without being attached to the results of his actions and to accept both success and failure with equanimity. I believe that this approach, which allowed Gandhi to attain some measure of inner peace and supported him as he developed and engaged in nonviolent social activism—where he often put his own life on the line—can help anyone who is engaging in service or social activism.

Melitta Rorty says that in her work as an advocate for people with type 1 diabetes, the philosophy of Karma Yoga, which she considers her path, supports her in the challenges she faces:

> For me, not being attached to a specific outcome is essential—I follow specific actions, but I never know what the outcome will be. Quite a number of people, after they have gotten a correct diagnosis and treatment, have told me that this literally saved their lives. But some people who I have coached are not willing to stand up to their doctors—to be their own best advocates within the medical system—and I have had to simply let go in those instances. Those situations are heartbreaking, and in two cases they rapidly developed horrific diabetic complications, which are preventable if correctly treated. But practicing Karma Yoga enables me to continue act in service to others, as I act for a greater good, without regard to personal gain or being attached to a particular outcome.[29]

As Melitta mentioned, for people who engage in acts of service and social activism, another aspect of Karma Yoga is taking your actions "without regard to personal gain." This means—in addition to letting go of expectations for the outcome of your work— you also let go of any personal expectations of receiving benefits, recognition, or even gratitude as a result of them. To enable you to maintain your equanimity as you serve others, your service must truly be "selfless service."

Obviously, it's hard to remain detached from results when you're fighting for a just cause, working for positive change, or standing up for what is right. But you can try your best, and the Gita says those efforts alone will be rewarding. Gandhi explains it this way:

> A beginning made is not wasted. Even a little effort along this path saves one from great danger. This is a royal road, easy to follow. It is the sovereign yoga. In following it, there is no fear of stumbling. Once a beginning is made, nothing will stand in our way.[30]

ACKNOWLEDGMENTS

Although I came up with the idea for this book before the pandemic, by the time I started writing it, the area in California where I live was locked down and I was in a bubble of two, just me and my husband, Brad. But throughout that year, as I worked alone in my little upstairs office with its window facing the old camphor tree, I often marveled at how, despite my physical isolation, there were so many people supporting me as I worked. Some were old friends, some were new friends, and some were friends I only know through email or Zoom. But all of them were very interesting people, with many different areas of expertise, and all gave generously of their time. I'm so grateful to you all:

Beth Frankl: There would be no book without you! In 2019 you asked me if I was interested in writing another book for Shambhala, this time by myself, something I hadn't even really considered before. And when I came up with the idea of writing a book about yoga for adapting to and accepting change—before the pandemic, mind you—you loved the idea immediately and supported me through the process of writing the proposal and then the book itself.

Richard Rosen: While I was writing the proposal, you gave me feedback on various ideas I was considering and guided me to a wide range of books that changed my thinking and my basic approach to various topics. And when I was writing the book, you were there when I had questions, and you helped me with the sections on breath awareness, pranayama, and impermanence.

Melitta Rorty: As my yoga study buddy from way back, as I researched my new book, you read many of the same things I was reading and met with me regularly over Zoom to discuss them. As someone who "lives" your yoga, you shared many of your personal stories with me about how yoga has helped you through the years. Then, when the final draft was done, you read almost the whole thing!

Ken Jackson and Carol Williams: My longtime friends who are both writers themselves, you were my very first readers, reviewing early drafts of chapters and making suggestions, and you encouraged me in the early days when I was sometimes beset with doubts.

Dr. Lynn Somerstein: A longtime yoga therapist and psychoanalyst, you shared your expertise especially generously with me, allowing me to pick your brain about anger, anxiety, depression, and grief, and you reviewed essential parts of the book.

Dr. Scott Lauzé: You inspired me more than I can say by sharing your thoughts with me about why mindfulness practices and Buddhist philosophy are so valuable for people dealing with emotional challenges and changed the way I thought about "negative" emotions.

Charlotte Bell: A longtime yoga teacher and practitioner of mindfulness meditation, you helped me with the section on mindfulness and shared your personal stories about how the practice has helped you and how you teach your own students. How glad I am we finally connected.

Barrie Risman: You not only did an amazing job at setting up the Canadian photo shoot for the book and being the sole model, but you also helped me with the sequences themselves, reviewed the chapter on yoga philosophy, and gave me feedback on other parts of the book that you read. And your friendship helped sustain me through what was such a difficult year for all of us.

Bonnie Maeda: I've always been inspired by the way you teach yoga for grief, but for the book you took the time to tell me more about your own experiences with grief as well as your tips for teaching yoga to others who are who are grieving. Thanks for being one of my teachers.

Jivana Heyman: You supported me as a fellow author, generously shared such honest and authentic stories about how yoga has helped you over the years, and reviewed my yoga philosophy chapter when I needed a reality check.

Beth Gibbs: Your lifelong dedication to yoga and the depth of your knowledge about areas of yoga I'm not very familiar with has always inspired me. For this book, I not only quoted you extensively, once again, but you came through with new personal stories about how yoga helped you through the ups and downs of your own life.

Sandy Blaine, Charissa Loftis, Robin Sturis, Erin Collins, Nina Rook, Jarvis Chen, Yoriko Matsumoto, Ram Rao, Cherie Hotchkiss, Patrice Priya Wagner, Elissa Rosenthal, Jill Satterfield, Amber Karnes, Ariel, Tracey, and "Jacqueline": Thanks to all of you for your stories, suggestions, tips, and insights about yoga and related topics.

Edwin F. Bryant and William K. Mahony: You generously answered some tricky questions I had about yoga philosophy. It was a privilege to be able to consult with you.

Éliane Excoffier and Cary Lawrence: I was worried about how to pull off a photo shoot during the pandemic, but the two of you, plus Barrie Risman who produced the photo shoot and was the model, were the best photo shoot team this author could hope for! Éliane, all your photographs of Barrie were not only beautiful and well organized, but you managed to complete the shoot in under the estimated time. Cary, you did a wonderful job of making sure the poses matched my specifications and that Barrie looked her best in every single one of them. You both combined a sincere enthusiasm for the project along with professionalism.

Brad Gibson: You not only were there every day for me to let me talk through what I was working on over lunch and dinner, but you carefully read every single word of the final draft of the book, identifying sections that weren't clear or were misleading. You'll even be reading this acknowledgments section for me. I know the book is a better one because of you.

Samantha Ripley: You were so patient and kind as you guided me through what for me are always the most challenging parts of writing a book—the copyediting and proofing phases.

APPENDIX
TIPS FOR STAYING SAFE

No one can guarantee you'll never hurt yourself while doing yoga. After all, no physical activity is risk free. You could hurt yourself walking your dog, taking care of your garden, or even just sitting at your desk. But there are some commonsense approaches you can take that will greatly reduce your chances of injuring yourself. And, as you'll see when you read through these guidelines, taking these approaches will also enable you to practice your yoga poses mindfully—paying attention to pain levels, breath, energy levels, and motivations for doing poses or not doing them—which is one of the aims of the asana practice.

I put together these nine guidelines a few years ago by consulting with a physical therapist, Shari Ser, and a medical doctor, Baxter Bell, both of whom are longtime teachers of yoga.

1. **Work with a teacher.** If you're taking a class, tell your teacher about any injuries, illnesses, conditions, or problems that might affect your ability to do certain poses or put you at risk. Your teacher can then help you figure out what you should not be doing and give you alternatives or at least understand why you're choosing to do something different at times. If you're practicing at home with an injury, illness, condition, or problem that might affect how you practice, consider taking a private lesson from a yoga therapist or experienced yoga teacher to help you choose the best poses for you to practice during this time.

2. **Pay attention to pain.** Learn to tell the difference between sensations that are potentially good for you, such as the healthy stretch of a tight muscle, and those that could be potentially injurious to you, such as overstretching a tendon or ligament,

or compressing structures to the point of injury. If you catch yourself moving into a painful or uncomfortable sensation that feels dangerous or that you are concerned about in any way, try backing out a bit, perhaps by letting go of a stretch or by using a prop. If you can't back out for some reason, come out of the pose and rest (see below). And keep in mind that the closer the pain is to a joint, the greater the potential there is for a problem.

3. **Listen to your breath.** Although your breath may come more quickly in demanding poses such as backbends or long-held standing poses, gasping for breath indicates you're overstressing yourself, so see if you can back out of the pose a bit, possibly by using a prop. If you can't back out for some reason or if doing that doesn't help you catch your breath, come out of the pose and rest (see below). Also, as you practice, notice if you are *holding* your breath because this is a possible sign you are becoming a bit fearful or anxious, or reacting to pain. If you realize you are reacting to pain, back out of the pose until the pain is gone or, if the pain stays, come out of the pose altogether. However, if you realize that you are just holding your breath, try to consciously relax your breathing.

4. **Rest if you need to.** If you feel you've reached your limit with your time in a pose, no matter what, come out and take a rest. Likewise, if you are suddenly sweating much more than normal, this may also be a sign that you're overstressing yourself, and you should take the same precautions. Some suggested ways to rest include:

   - If you're doing supine poses (on your back), rest in Savasana.
   - If you're doing prone poses (on your belly), rest in Prone Savasana.
   - If you're doing seated poses on the floor, rest in Easy Sitting pose (Sukasana), where you sit with crossed legs, or in Thunderbolt pose (Vajrasana), where you sit on your heels.
   - If you're seated on a chair, come into seated Mountain pose.
   - If you're doing standing poses, rest in Mountain pose.
   - If you are doing inverted poses, come down into Child's pose.

   If you feel like you just can't finish the rest of a class, either let the teacher know so they can give you a resting pose to finish with or just lie down in a comfortable Savasana. If you're practicing on your own at home and can't finish a sequence, choose any resting pose you like. Just don't stop in the middle of a practice without cooling down.

5. **Stay balanced.** If you are weak or have trouble with balance, use props, such as a chair or the wall, to stabilize yourself so you don't fall over and can practice with confidence. You can practice with your back to a wall, with one foot on the wall in standing poses, or with a hand on the wall in certain poses. If you know you have problems with balance, come to class early and stake out a place next to the wall so the wall will always be there when you need it. And if you're practicing at home, make sure your practice space has a wall that you can use for support when needed.

6. **Use props.** Even if you have not been specially instructed to use a prop and you know that it is important for your safety (to keep you from overstretching or falling or to use as padding for sensitive areas), go ahead and use it. And if you know you typically need a certain prop, such as a block or blanket, have one ready at your side before class or your home practice begins.

7. **Resist peer pressure.** If your class is doing a pose that you feel is beyond your capabilities or that you just aren't ready for, just don't do it. Ask your teacher for an alternative or take a resting pose. Or you can just watch the others do the pose and learn through observation. If your class is consistently too challenging for you, look for another class that fits your level of ability, such as an eight-week introductory series for beginners, an Accessible Yoga class, a class that is designed specifically for people like you, or even just a class in a different style of yoga. If you're practicing at home, you might still have imaginary peers that you're trying to keep up with, so if you notice that about yourself, tell them to get lost. After all, one of the wonderful things about practicing on your own is that no one can see you!

8. **Only do inverted poses if they're okay for you.** Inverted poses are contraindicated for people who have uncontrolled high blood pressure, for those who are having eye problems, such as glaucoma or detached retina, and for other conditions. And if you are having neck problems, please refrain from practicing Headstand, Shoulderstand, and Plow. If you have no contraindications, the supported inverted poses shown in this book are gentle and generally safe. But if you want to learn the more active inverted poses, such as Headstand and Shoulderstand, start by finding a special class, series, or workshop that is designed to introduce you step by step to the inverted poses, so you can learn to practice these poses safely, under the careful guidance of an experienced teacher.

9. Talk to your doctor and/or physical therapist. If you have had a surgery or if you have a medical condition or an injury, before you return to your yoga class or home practice, ask your doctor or physical therapist explicitly about which physical actions are safe for you and which are not. Don't wait for your medical professionals to tell you! Some medical professionals don't really know what a yoga class is like, even while they recommend "yoga." Some imagine it's just a gentle stretching session and might not even consider that you could be going upside down, twisting yourself like a pretzel, or sweating from a vigorous practice. So when you are checking in about whether you're ready to practice yoga yet, consider bringing a yoga book with you so you can show the doctor or physical therapist the types of poses you normally do. You should also ask some specific questions, such as:

- Can I go upside down for long holds or even short ones?
- Can I twist my spine or round my spine forward, backward, or side to side?
- Can I cross my legs?
- Can I put pressure on this or that part of my body, such as my knees or wrists?
- Can I stand on one leg?
- Can I practice in bare feet?
- Is my recovery from a serious illness, such as cancer or heart disease, at a place where I can safely increase my physical activity?
- Is it safe for me to do a vigorous practice that makes me sweat and exert myself? Is it okay for me to hold standing poses for long periods of time that require endurance and strength?
- Is it all right to stretch an injured tendon, ligament, or muscle now?
- Would any of the medicine I am taking interfere with my practicing by making me dizzy, unfocused, distracted, off-balance, or sleepy?
- How long should I wait before returning to class or home practice? After surgery, how long do I wait before it is safe to stretch the area where my incision or scar is? If I have had a joint replacement or repair, such as a hip or knee, is there a limit to my range of motion in certain directions that I should honor?

It's your one and only precious body, so it makes sense to be cautious and follow the recommendations you receive.

NOTES

Chapter 1: Introduction

1. T. K. V. Desikachar, *The Heart of Yoga: Developing a Personal Practice* (Rochester, VT: Inner Traditions International, 1995), 12.
2. Juan Mascaro, trans., *The Bhagavad Gita* (New York: Penguin, 1962), 12.
3. Robert Wright, *Why Buddhism Is True: The Science and Philosophy of Meditation and Enlightenment* (New York: Simon and Schuster, 2017), 233.
4. B. K. S. Iyengar, *Light on the Yoga Sutras of Patanjali* (London: George Allen & Unwin, 1966), 105.
5. Edwin F. Bryant, *The Yoga Sutras of Patanjali* (New York: North Point Press, 2009), 189.
6. Bryant, *The Yoga Sutras of Patanjali*, 189.
7. Stanley B. Klein, Theresa E. Robertson, and Andrew W. Delton, "Facing the Future: Memory as an Evolved System for Planning Future Acts," *Memory and Cognition* 38, no. 1 (January 2010): 13–22.
8. Georg Feuerstein, trans., *The Bhagavad Gita: A New Translation* (Boston, MA: Shambhala Publications, 2014), 109.
9. Georg Feuerstein, *The Yoga Tradition: Its History, Literature, Philosophy and Practice* (Prescott, AZ: Hohm Press, 1998), 7.
10. Mascaro, *Bhagavad Gita*, 29.
11. Wright, *Why Buddhism Is True*, 253.
12. Bryant, *The Yoga Sutras of Patanjali*, 360.

Chapter 2: Coping with Change

1. Richard Rosen, *The Yoga of Breath* (Boulder: Shambhala Publications, 2002), 122.

Chapter 3: Stress Management for When You're Stressed

1. Robert Wright, *Why Buddhism Is True: The Science and Philosophy of Meditation and Enlightenment* (New York: Simon and Schuster, 2017), 117.
2. Wright, *Why Buddhism Is True*, 119.
3. Scott Lauzé, personal correspondence.

Chapter 4: Moving Through Anger, Anxiety, and Depression

1. Jon Kabat-Zinn, *Full Catastrophe Living: Using the Wisdom of Your Body and Mind to Face Stress, Pain, and Illness* (New York: Bantam Books, 2013), 412.
2. Kang Seon Lee et al., "Ramped Up Fight-or-Flight Response Points to History of Warfare for Humans and Chimps," *Science Daily*, April 19, 2018.
3. Lynn Somerstein, "Anger and Yoga: Interview with Dr. Lynn Somerstein," *Yoga for Healthy Aging Blog*, February 8, 2021, https://www.yogafortimesofchange.com/anger-and-yoga-interview-with-dr-lynn.
4. Lauzé, personal correspondence.
5. Sharon Salzberg, *Real Change: Mindfulness to Heal Ourselves and the World* (New York: Flatiron Books, 2020), 59.
6. Charissa Loftis, "Three Steps for Working with Anger," *Yoga for Healthy Aging Blog*, June 21, 2017, https://www.yogafortimesofchange.com/three-steps-for-working-with-anger.
7. Lauzé, personal correspondence.
8. Jarvis Chen, personal correspondence.
9. Beth Gibbs, "Understanding and Dealing with Anger," *Yoga for Healthy Aging Blog*, May 16, 2017, https://www.yogafortimesofchange.com/understanding-and-dealing-with-anger.
10. Somerstein, "Anger and Yoga: Interview with Dr. Lynn Somerstein."
11. Nina Rook, "Comfort with Uncertainty," *Yoga for Healthy Aging Blog*, November 1, 2016, https://www.yogafortimesofchange.com/comfort-with-uncertainty.
12. Lauzé, personal correspondence.
13. Tara Brach, *Radical Acceptance: Embracing Your Life with the Heart of a Buddha* (New York: Bantam Dell, 2003), 166.
14. Lynn Somerstein, "Anxiety and Yoga: An Interview with Dr. Lynn Somerstein," *Yoga Pit*, January 23, 2021, https://yoga-pit.com/2021/01/25/anxiety-and-yoga-interview-with-dr-lynn-somerstein.

15. Rook, "Comfort with Uncertainty."

16. Jivana Heyman, personal correspondence.

17. Lauzé, personal correspondence.

18. Timothy McCall, *Yoga as Medicine: The Yogic Prescription for Health and Healing* (New York: Bantam Books, 2007), 553.

19. Melitta Rorty, personal correspondence.

20. Lynn Somerstein, "Depression and Yoga: An Interview with Dr. Lynn Somerstein," *Accessible Yoga Blog*, June 12, 2020, http://accessibleyoga.blogspot.com/2020/06/depression-and-yoga-interview-with-dr.html.

21. Somerstein, "Depression and Yoga: An Interview with Dr. Lynn Somerstein."

22. Quoted in *Yoga as Medicine*, 558.

23. Quoted in *Yoga as Medicine*, 559.

24. Jack Kornfield, "The Sacred Pause," JackKornfield.com, accessed September 15, 2021, https://jackkornfield.com/the-sacred-pause.

25. Yoriko Matsumoto, "Serendipity: Discovering Yoga for Depression," *Yoga for Healthy Aging Blog*, June 6, 2017, https://www.yogafortimesofchange.com/serendipity-discovering-yoga-for/

26. Edwin F. Bryant, *The Yoga Sutras of Patanjali* (New York: North Point Press, 2009), 243

Chapter 5: Moving Through Grief

1. Bonnie Maeda, "Grief and Yoga: An Interview with Bonnie Maeda, RN," *Yoga for Healthy Aging Blog*, October 5, 2020, https://www.yogafortimesofchange.com/grief-and-yoga-interview-with-bonnie.

2. Erin Collins, "A Hospice Nurse on Yoga for Grief," *Yoga for Healthy Aging Blog*, https://www.yogafortimesofchange.com/a-hospice-nurse-on-yoga-for-grief.

3. Sharon Salzberg, *Real Change: Mindfulness to Heal Ourselves and the World* (New York: Flatiron Books, 2020), 98.

4. Maeda, "Grief and Yoga: An Interview with Bonnie Maeda, RN."

5. Christopher D. Wallis, *Tantra Illuminated: The Philosophy, History and Practice of a Timeless Tradition* (Petaluma, CA: Mattamayūra Press, 2012), 65.

6. Jivana Heyman, "The Eye of the Storm," *Yoga for Healthy Aging Blog*, November 8, 2017, https://www.yogafortimesofchange.com/the-eye-of-storm.

7. Heyman, "The Eye of the Storm."

8. Robin Sturis, "Yoga for Grief, Anger, and Shame," *Yoga for Healthy Aging Blog*, June 13, 2017, https://www.yogafortimesofchange.com/yoga-for-grief-anger-and-shame.

9. Maeda, "Grief and Yoga: An Interview with Bonnie Maeda, RN."

10. Sturis, "Yoga for Grief, Anger, and Shame."

11. Maeda, "Grief and Yoga: An Interview with Bonnie Maeda, RN."

12. Collins, "A Hospice Nurse on Yoga for Grief."

13. Maeda, "Grief and Yoga: An Interview with Bonnie Maeda, RN."

Chapter 6: Adapting to Physical Changes

1. Ariel, personal correspondence.

2. Edwin F. Bryant, *The Yoga Sutras of Patanjali* (New York: North Point Press, 2009), 286.

Chapter 7: Being Present

1. Christopher D. Wallis, *Tantra Illuminated: The Philosophy, History and Practice of a Timeless Tradition* (Petaluma, CA: Mattamayūra Press, 2012), 139.

2. Wallis, *Tantra Illuminated*, 139.

3. Georg Feuerstein, *The Yoga Tradition: Its History, Literature, Philosophy and Practice* (Prescott, AZ: Hohm Press, 1998), 137.

4. Sally Kempton, *Meditation for the Love of It: Enjoying Your Own Deepest Experience* (Boulder, CO: Sounds True, 2011), 100.

5. See Richard Rosen, *The Yoga of Breath* (Boulder: Shambhala Publications, 2002) and *Pranayama beyond the Fundamentals* (Boulder: Shambhala Publications, 2006); B. K. S. Iyengar, *Light on Pranayama* (London: Unwin Paperbacks, 1983); and Nina Zolotow and Baxter Bell, *Yoga for Healthy Aging: A Guide to Lifelong Well-Being* (Boulder: Shambhala Publications, 2017).

6. Jill Satterfield, "Spiritual Sanity," *Yoga for Healthy Aging Blog*, August 14, 2014, https://www.yogafortimesofchange.com/spiritual-sanity.

7. Scott Lauzé, personal correspondence.

8. Wallis, *Tantra Illuminated*, 105.

9. Edwin F. Bryant, *The Yoga Sutras of Patanjali* (New York: North Point Press, 2009), 139.

10. Kempton, *Meditation for the Love of It*, 73.

11. Lynn Somerstein, "Friday Q&A: Depression, Medication, and Meditation," *Yoga for Healthy Aging* (blog), June 12, 2015, www.yogafortimesofchange.com/friday-q-depression-medication-and/.

12. Lauzé, personal correspondence.

13. Kempton, *Meditation for the Love of It*, 96.

14. Patrice Priya Wagner, "What's So Good About Meditating, Part 2: Making Friends with Your Mind," *Accessible Yoga Blog*, March 4, 2020, https://accessibleyoga.blog-spot.com/2020/03/whats-so-good-about-meditation-part-1.html.

15. Elissa C. Rosenthal, "A Caregiving Warrior Exhales with Yoga Practices," *Accessible Yoga Blog*, December 6, 2019, https://accessibleyoga.blogspot.com/2019/12/a-caregiving-warrior-exhales-with-yoga.html.

16. Wallis, *Tantra Illuminated*, 129.

17. David Gelles, "How to Meditate," *New York Times*, accessed September 16, 2021, https://www.nytimes.com/guides/well/how-to-meditate.

18. Charlotte Bell, personal correspondence.

19. Kempton, *Meditation for the Love of It*, 155.

20. Bell, personal correspondence.

21. Sharon Salzberg, *Real Change: Mindfulness to Heal Ourselves and the World* (New York: Flatiron Books, 2020), 69.

22. Wallis, *Tantra Illuminated*, 53.

23. Bell, personal correspondence.

Chapter 8: Making Peace with Change

1. Nina Rook, "Comfort with Uncertainty," *Yoga for Healthy Aging Blog*, November 1, 2016, https://www.yogafortimesofchange.com/comfort-with-uncertainty.

2. Edwin Bryant, personal correspondence.

3. Edwin F. Bryant, *The Yoga Sutras of Patanjali* (New York: North Point Press, 2009), 179.

4. Georg Feuerstein, *The Yoga Tradition: Its History, Literature, Philosophy and Practice* (Prescott, AZ: Hohm Press, 1998), 254.

5. Sally Kempton, *Meditation for the Love of It: Enjoying Your Own Deepest Experience* (Boulder, CO: Sounds True, 2011), 311.

6. Jivana Heyman, personal correspondence.

7. Juan Mascaro, trans., *The Bhagavad Gita* (New York: Penguin, 1962), 10.

8. Barrie Risman, personal correspondence.

9. Barbara Stoler Miller, *Yoga: Discipline of Freedom* (New York: Bantam Books, 1998), 78.

10. Christopher D. Wallis, *Tantra Illuminated: The Philosophy, History and Practice of a Timeless Tradition* (Petaluma, CA: Mattamayūra Press, 2012), 65.

11. Sharon Salzberg, *Real Change: Mindfulness to Heal Ourselves and the World* (New York: Flatiron Books, 2020), 52.

12. B. K. S. Iyengar, *Light on Life: The Yoga Journey to Wholeness, Inner Peace, and Ultimate Freedom* (Emmaus, PA: Rodale, 2005), 256.

13. Gandhi, *Young India*, May 20, 1926.

14. Wallis, *Tantra Illuminated*, 361.

15. Risman, personal correspondence.

16. Lauzé, personal correspondence.

17. Lauzé, personal correspondence.

18. Bryant, *The Yoga Sutras of Patanjali*, 129.

19. Stephen Cope, *The Wisdom of Yoga: A Seeker's Guide to Extraordinary Living* (New York: Bantam Books, 2006), 180.

20. Pema Chödrön, *When Things Fall Apart: Heart Advice for Difficult Times* (Boulder, CO: Shambhala, 2016), 26.

21. Lauzé, personal correspondence.

22. "Yoga Sutra 1.33," Yoga International website, accessed September 17, 2021, https://yogainternational.com/article/view/yoga-sutra-1-33-translation-and-commentary.

23. Mahatma Gandhi, "The 'Quit India' Speech," Bombay Sarvodaya Mandal/Gandhi Book Centre, accessed September 16, 2021, https://www.mkgandhi.org/speeches/qui.htm.

24. Ram Rao, "Forgiveness (Kshama)," *Yoga for Healthy Aging Blog*, November 12, 2014, https://www.yogafortimesofchange.com/forgiveness-kshama.

25. Stephen Mitchell, trans., *Bhagavad Gita: A New Translation* (New York: Harmony Books, 2000), 62.

26. Mitchell, *Bhagavad Gita*, 55.

27. Georg Feuerstein, *The Deeper Dimension of Yoga: Theory and Practice* (Boston and London: Shambhala, 2003), 269.

28. Mahatma Gandhi, *The Bhagavad Gita according to Gandhi* (Berkeley: Berkeley Hills Books, 2000), 148

29. Melitta Rorty, "Melitta Rorty on Service, Social Activism, and Yoga," *Accessible Yoga Blog*, September 5, 2019, https://accessibleyoga.blogspot.com/2019/09/melitta-rorty-on-service-social.html.

30. Gandhi, *The Bhagavad Gita according to Gandhi*, 45

INDEX

Page numbers in *italics* indicate images.

Abhinava Gupta, 234

Accessible Yoga, 169, 173, 267
  Heyman and, 85, 155, 182, 250

action, yoga of, 172, 248–49, 254–59

Adho Mukha Vrksasana, 93

Advaita Vedanta, 227, 228–29

aesthetic rapture, 212

afflictions (*kleshas*), 5, 6, 233

ahamkara (ego), 233

ahimsa, 139–40, 169, 203, 246,
    251, 258

Alternate Nostril Breath, 190, 191, 194

anger, 90–101
  moving through, 92–97
  sequences for, 98–101

anxiety, 102–14
  breath practice and, 190, 191
  as future oriented, 187
  moving through, 104–10, 212
  physical experiences of, 103–4, 109, 240
  professional help with, 87, 104
  sequences for, 111–14
  stress and, 69, 70

aparigraha (non-possessiveness), 140, 241

Ardha Adho Mukha Svanasana. *See* Half
    Downward-Facing Dog

Ardha Chandrasana, 177

Ardha Halasana, 23, 26, 27

Ardha Matseyendrasana, 176

Ardha Padmasana, 220

Ardha Viparita Karani. *See* Easy Inverted
    pose

arjava (honesty), 171, 236–42

Arms Overhead pose, 49, 51, 121
  Reclined, 100, 120, 129, 181
  in sequences, 46, 163
  as vinyasa, 50, 123

asanas. *See* poses

asmita (ego), 233

asteya (non-stealing), 140

attachment, 4–8, 140, 172
  cultivating non-, 242–44, 256–57

attraction, 4–6, 241

Aurobindo, 257

aversion, 6, 68, 87, 91, 241. *See also* dvesa
    (aversion)

backbends
    contraindications for, 106, 148
    for depression, 89, 120, 130
    grieving and, 148, 151
    supported, 125, 130, 132–33
bahya kumbhaka. *See* breath practices:
    retention
balancing, 45, 267
Balasana. *See* Child's pose
bed-bound yoga, 36, 173, 179, 181,
    183, 195
Bell, Baxter, 265
Bell, Charlotte, 154, 213–15, 216, 217, 219
Bensen, Herbert, 76
Bhagavad Gita, 256
    on equanimity, 3, 6, 8, 9, 10, 172, 224, 251
    on eternal, 226, 227, 230–31
    on karma yoga, 254–59
Bhramari pranayama, 193, 194
Blaine, Sandy, 48, 89
blood pressure regulation, 24–25
Boat pose, 176
Body Positive Yoga, 169
body scans, 35, 38, 173, 215
Bow pose, Supported, 128
Brach, Tara, 96, 102, 103, 213
brahmacarya (sexual restraint), 140
brahmavihara (divine abodes), 245
brains, 212, 231
breath awareness, 17–23, 63
    for anxiety, 107
    in asana, 172, 266
    for grief, 157
    for insomnia, 56
    in meditation, 154, 156, 208–9
    positions for, 18–21, 35, 38

    as self-inquiry, 240
    techniques for, 21–23
breath practices, 189–200
    for anger, 93, 94, 95
    for anxiety, 105, 106, 108
    for balancing, 11, 190, 191, 194, 198
    basics of, 194–96
    for being present, 12, 188
    calming, 89, 105, 197
    choosing, 62–63
    contraindications for, 18, 94, 106, 190,
        194, 196
    for depression, 121
    Equal Ratio Breath, 198
    exhalation focused, 84, 101, 130, 133, 193, 197
    as gateway to meditation, 189–91
    inhalation focused, 121, 125, 193
    for insomnia, 56
    for letting go, 243
    moving with (*see* vinyasas)
    nervous system regulation and, 191–94
    observation of (*see* breath awareness)
    postures for, 219–21
    retention, 23, 191, 194, 209, 229
    Skull Shining Breath, 198–200
    stimulating, 63, 131, 191, 193, 198–200
    for stress, 73–74
    timing for, 196
Bridge pose, 50, 93, 128
    Supported (*see* Supported Bridge)
    vinyasa, 122, 123
buddhi (wisdom mind), 237
Buddhism, 202, 203, 204, 230, 231, 245
Bryant, Edwin, 227
    Patanjali interpreted by, 5, 6, 10, 139, 172, 245
    Patanjali translated by, 244, 246

Camel pose (Ustrasana), 178

Cat-Cow, 50, 93, 97, 124

   in sequences, 53, 127

chairs, 181–82, 220

   Child's pose with, 182

   cultivating awareness in, 18–19, 43

   forward bends sitting in, 58, 95, 107,

      114, 150–51

   forward bends leaning on, 39,

      113, 158

   injury recovery using, 92, 169–70

   Savasana with, 30, 31, 128

   Shoulderstand with, 23

   Sun Salutations with, 162, 163

chanakara (aesthetic rapture), 212

Chandogya Upanishad, 230

change

   accepting, 12, 200–201, 223–26

   coping skills for, 15–63

   exercises to experience, 226

   grief and, 143–44

   societal, 2, 67, 143–44

   unhealthy coping strategies for, 15

   yoga philosophy of, 2–4, 8–13, 223–25

   See also present, being in

Chen, Jarvis, 93, 95

chest-opening poses, 119, 120, 129, 164–67.

   See also backbends

Child's pose, 99, 113

   resting in, 161, 266

   Supported (see Supported Child's pose)

   in chair, 182

Chödrön, Pema, 246–47

Classical Yoga, 227–28

   ego in, 233

   eight limbs of, 75–76, 190, 203

   yamas in, 139–40

   See also Yoga Sutras (Patanjali)

Cobbler's pose. See Reclined Cobbler's

   pose

Cobra pose, at wall, 180, 182

Cole, Roger, 24

Collins, Erin, 143, 145, 153, 157

compassion, 141, 211, 247–49, 257. See also

   karuna (compassion)

concentration, 72–73

   asana as, 164

   mantra as, 155–56

   meditation as, 155–56, 202–3, 208–13, 251

   mindfulness vs., 213

   pranayama as, 188, 189–91

Cope, Stephen, 245

Corpse pose. See Savasana

Cow-Face pose, 121, 129, 177

   Standing Half-, 52, 166

Crescent Moon pose, 52

Crocodile pose. See Prone Savasana

Dancer's pose, 182

Darjeeling Limited, The (film), 242–43, 244

depression, 115–36

   meditation and, 205, 212

   moving through, 119–26, 129–34

   professional help with, 87, 117

   rajasic, 129–36

   sequences for, 127–28, 135–36

   stress and, 119

   tamasic, 117–28

Desikachar, T. K. V., 2–3, 246, 249, 250

Desk Forward Bend, 95, 107–8, 151

dharana. See concentration

discernment (tarka), 234–36

Downward-Facing Dog, 51, 93, 96, 161
    in chair Sun Salutations, 162, *163*
    Half (*see* Half Downward-Facing Dog)
    One-Legged, *99*
    in sequences, *47, 99, 111, 136, 159*
    Supported, 24, 27
    at wall, 178
drishti. *See* gaze
Dropped-Knee Lunge, 53, *128*
dualism, 227–28
dvesa (aversion), 6, 68, 87, 91, 241

Eagle pose, modifications of, 177
Easy Inverted pose, 114, 121, 130, 132, 134, 136
    in sequences, *27, 84, 167*
Easy Seated Twist, 158
Easy Sitting Forward Bend, Supported, *39, 113, 158*
Easy Sitting pose, *19*, 177, 219
    resting in, 161, 266
    See also Reclined Crossed-Legs pose
ego, 233
emotions
    accepting, 231–34
    inquiry into, 236–42
    meditating on, 13, 203–4, 210–13, 216–17
    painful, 85–90, 137–41, 241, 245
    stress and, 68–70, 87–89
    See also anger; anxiety; depression; grief
empathy, cultivation of, 203–4, 211
enlightenment vs. equanimity, 9–10
Equal Ratio Breath, 198
    as balancing, 190, 191, 194
    in sequences, 81
equanimity, 9–10, 211, 250–52, 256–57
eternal, 226–31

ethics. *See* yamas (guiding principles)
evolutionary psychology, 231
exercise, 59, 76. *See also* poses
Extended Side-Angle pose (Utthita
    Parsvakonasana), *47*, 177, *182*
Extending the Exhalation, 23, 56, 84,
    101, 197
exteroception, 42–43

fatigue, 156–59
fear, 92, 102–14
    moving through, 104–10
    physical experiences of, 103–4
    sequences for, 111–14
feelings. *See* emotions
Feuerstein, Georg, 9, 190, 228, 257
fight-flight-or-freeze response, 87–88
    amygdala and, 102, 138
    anger and, 90, 92
    anxiety and, 102, 104
    breathing and, 192–94, 199
    depression and, 115–16, 119
    inversions for, 93
    as physical tension, 48
    stress and, 68–69, 70
forgiveness, 141, 155, 252–54. *See also*
    kshama (forgiveness)
forward bends, 89
    for anxiety, 105, 107, 113–14
    contraindications for, 122, 131
    Seated (in chair), 58, 95, 107, 114, *150–51*
    Sitting (on floor), *39, 113, 158*
    Standing (*see* Standing Forward Bend)
friendship, 238
    unconditional, 73, 203, 211, 246–47
Full Catastrophe Living (Kabat-Zinn), 85–86

future, attachment to, 6–8, 102, 187, 241.
   See also present, being in

Gandhi, Mohandas, 139, 236, 251, 257, 258, 259
Garudasana, 177
gaze, 43, 62, 121, 130, 165
   in meditation, 207, 209
Gensen, Mumon, 1
Gibbs, Beth, 11, 94, 144, 156, 160, 236, 237
Gibson, Brad (husband), ix–x, 1–2, 15, 28, 66,
   68, 241
Gomukasana, 121, 129, 177
gratitude practices, 203, 211–12, 240
grief, 143–67
   change and, 5
   complexity of, 143–46
   contraindications for, 148
   eternal and, 230–31
   sequences for, 152, 156–67
   supporting others through, 154–55
   witnessing, 147, 148–56, 211
guided meditation, 73, 203, 212
   for relaxation, 57, 76, 221
   yoga nidra, 61, 73, 157, 164
gunas (qualities), 118, 254

Half Downward-Facing Dog, 49, 183
   in sequences, 52, 78, 82, 111, 135
Half Lord of the Fishes pose, 176
Half Lotus, 219–20, 221
Half Moon pose, 177
Half Pyramid pose, 78
hands, focusing on, 121, 130, 135
Handstand (Adho Mukha Vrksasana), 93, 96
   modifications to, 181, 184
Hariharananda, 245

Hatha yoga, 204, 224, 227–29
Hatha Yoga Pradipika, 171, 236, 253
Headstand (Sirsasana), 93, 183, 267
health issues. *See* modifications
Heart of Yoga, The (Desikachar), 2–3, 246,
   249, 250
Hero pose (Virasana), 19, 219
Heyman, Jivana, 90, 91, 230
   Accessible Yoga and, 85, 182, 250
   on anxiety, 109, 110, 240, 156
   on grief, 149, 153, 155
Hinduism, 230
hip openers, 54, 106, 160
honesty, 171, 236–42. *See also* arjava (honesty)
Hotchkiss, Cherie, 173
householders, 255

illness. *See* modifications
impermanence. *See* change
injury. *See* modifications
insomnia, 55–61, 217
   techniques to counter, 33, 36, 56–58
Integral Yoga, 174
interoception, 43–44, 215
inversions, supported. *See* supported
   inversions
Iyengar, B. K. S., 122, 132, 173
   on pranayama, 189, 196
   on yamas, 235, 247
Iyengar yoga, 50, 130, 174, 194

Jainism, 230
joy, 203, 211, 249–50

Kabat-Zinn, Jon, 85–86
kaivalya (aloneness), 228

Kapalabhati, 191, 193, 198–200. *See also* Skull
    Shining Breath
karma yoga, 254–59
Karnes, Amber, 169
karuna (compassion), 141, 211, 247–49, 257
Kempton, Sally, 191, 228, 242, 252
    on meditation, 205, 208, 216, 229
kindness, 140, 211, 244–52
King, Martin Luther, Jr., 139, 258
kleshas (afflictions), 5, 6, 233
Kornfield, Jack, 137
Krishnamacharya, Tirumalai, 173
kshama (forgiveness), 141, 155, 252–54
kumbhaka. *See* breath practices: retention

Lasater, Judith Hanson, 28, 36
Lauzé, Scott, 91, 92, 248
    on acceptance, 223, 225, 254
    on fight-flight-or-freeze, 70, 102, 115–16, 138
    on meditation, 201, 205
    on self-inquiry, 139, 238, 239–40
    on skillful responding, 139, 238
    on thought, 231, 232
Leg Stretches
    Reclined 49, 51, 54, 82–83, 100, 180
    Standing, 180, 183
Legs Up the Wall, 65, 74, 77, 79, 145
    as counterpose, 26
    as final pose, 59, 161, 167
    in sequences, 79, 101, 114, 136
    Supported, 23, 25, 27, 121, 132
letting go, 155, 234–54
Libby, Dan, 70
Light on Life (Iyengar), 247
Light on Pranayama (Iyengar), 196
Light on the Yoga Sutras (Iyengar), 189

Locust pose, 176, 182
    Standing, 52, 121, 125, 129, 166
    Supported, 128
Loftis, Charissa, 91, 93, 96, 97, 141, 248–49
Lotus pose, 219
loving-kindness, 73, 203, 211, 246–47, 253.
    See also maitri (loving-kindness);
    metta (loving-kindness)
Lunge
    in chair Sun Salutations, 163
    Dropped-Knee, 53, 128
    lying down, 20
    See also Savasana; prone poses;
    supine poses

Maeda, Bonnie, 143, 145, 146, 148, 156, 157, 161
    personal grief of, 144, 154, 160
maitri (loving-kindness), 73, 203, 211,
    246–47, 253
Makrasana. *See* Prone Savasana
Mandela, Nelson, 139, 258
mantra, 56, 155–56, 188, 251
    examples of, 209–10
    positions for, 35, 38
    See also concentration
Marichi's pose (Marichyasana), 3, 176
Marjaryasana Bitilasana. *See* Cat-Cow
Mascaro, Juan, 6, 8, 224, 230
Matsumoto, Yoriko, 138
McCall, Timothy, 116, 121, 130
meditation, 12–13, 72–73, 188, 200–221
    basics of, 200–202, 205–8
    choosing, 204–5
    concentration, 155–56, 202–3, 208–10, 251
    contraindications for, 106, 122, 131, 205
    on daily life, 212, 218–19

guided, 57, 73, 212

mindfulness, 153–54, 204–5, 208, 213–19, 252

nonattachment in, 243–44

postures for, 207, 219–21

pranayama as prep for, 189–91

Savasana as, 28–29, 73

self-inquiry in, 238

for training mind and heart, 203–4, 210–13

transitions for, 208

on universal kindness, 211, 249, 250, 253

Meditation for the Love of It (Kempton), 191, 205, 208, 228, 242, 252

metta (loving-kindness), 73, 203, 211, 246–47, 253

Miller, Barbara Stoler, 233

mind, 237

overidentifying with, 231–34

See also thoughts

mindfulness. *See under* meditation

Mitchell, Stephen, 226, 255

mobility issues. *See* modifications

Modern Postural Yoga, 224

modifications, xiii–xiv, 160–61, 169–85, 265–68

of pose orientations, 179–84

props for, 172, 178

simplifying, 175–77

using a wall, 177–78, 182–83

visualization as, 173

wisdom of, 171–72

Mountain pose, 46, 98, 159, 163, 166

breath awareness in, 18

meditating in, 221

resting in, 161, 266

Sideways, 53

Moyer, Donald, 40–41, 45

mudita (sympathetic joy), 211, 249–50

Nadi Shodhana, 190, 191, 194

Natarajasana, 182

Navasana, 176

nervous system, 66–71, 191–94. *See also* fight-flight-or-freeze response

Nhat Hanh, Thich, 95

nonattachment, 242–44, 256–57

non-dualism, 228–29

non-possessiveness, 140

non-stealing, 140

nonviolence, 139–40, 169, 246, 258

Gandhi on, 236, 251

See also loving-kindness

Noose pose (Pasasana), 178

One-Legged Downward-Facing Dog, 99

osteoarthritis, 170

Padmasana, 220

pandemic, 2, 5, 6, 8, 15, 28, 90, 239

adapting to, 88, 109, 224–25

parinamavada (continual change), 3

Pasasana, 178

past, attachment to, 5–6, 187. *See also* present, being in

Patanjali. *See* Yoga Sutras (Patanjali)

Phalankasana, 162, 182

physical changes. *See* modifications

Plank pose (Phalankasana), 162, 182

Plow pose, 267

Supported, 23, 26, 27

poses, 40–47
  for balance, 11
  breath in, 172, 266
  compassion and, 249
  contraindications for, 27, 48, 94, 106, 122,
    131, 148, 265–68
  demanding, 93, 96, 106, 122
  for depression, 120–21, 122–25, 127–28,
    129–33, 135–36
  dynamic (see vinyasas)
  emotions and, 138–39, 234
  foundations of, 175–76
  frustrating, 94
  gentle, 175
  for grief, 147, 152, 156–67
  home practice, 59–61, 90, 184, 195, 206
  letting go in, 244
  for meditation and pranayama, 219–21
  mindfulness in, 12, 41–45, 172
  modifications for (see modifications)
  orientation of, 179–84
  as preparation for relaxation, 73, 74
  resting between, 161, 266
  safety in, 265–68
  self-inquiry in, 238
  sequences of (see sequences)
  sequencing, 27, 36–37, 42, 76–77, 161,
    184–85, 190
  stimulating, 77
  visualization of, 173
  See also restorative yoga; stretching; specific
    poses
positivity, cultivating, 235, 244
pranayama. See breath practices
Pranayama beyond the Fundamentals (Rosen),
  196

pratipaksha bhavana (cultivate the opposite),
  244, 247, 249, 250, 253
present, being in, 187–221, 244
  forgiveness and, 253
  meditations for, 200–221
  pranayama for, 189–219, 219–21
prone poses, 150–51, 180, 182–83
Prone Savasana, 32, 39, 105, 108, 150, 266
Prone Twist (Supta Bharadvajasana), 20
  Supported, 39, 81, 152
proprioception, 44–45, 164–65, 215
props, 172, 178–79. See also restorative yoga;
  specific supported poses
Pyramid pose, 178
  Half, 78

Radical Acceptance (Brach), 102, 103, 213
Rao, Padma, 141, 252
Rao, Ram, 42, 141, 241, 252
Real Change (Salzberg), 91, 216, 218, 233
Reclined Arms Overhead pose, 100, 120,
  129, 181
Reclined Cobbler's pose, 20, 39, 58, 80, 125, 151
  Supported, 36, 158
Reclined Crossed-Legs pose, 38, 58, 80, 151, 158
Reclined Leg Stretches (Supta
  Padangusthasana), 49, 51, 180
  in sequences, 54, 82–83, 100
reclined poses, 151–52, 180, 221
  contraindications for, 106
  as modifications, 181
Reclined Twist, 54, 120, 128, 129
Relax and Renew (Lasater), 28, 36
relaxation, 57
  distraction vs., 72
  meditations for, 203, 212

response, 16, 21, 25, 71, 76, 196, 201
sleep vs., 28
troubleshooting, 61–63
Relaxation pose. *See* Savasana
Relaxation Response, The (Bensen), 76
religion, 230
resentment, 92
rest-and-digest state, 16, 60, 71, 72, 192
Restorative Savasana, 31
restorative yoga, 36–39
contraindications for, 122, 131
for insomnia, 57–58
modifications for, 183
for stress, 74, 80–81
timing of, 38–39
See also reclined and supported postures
Restore and Rebalance (Lasater), 36
right action, 254–59
Risman, Barrie, xiv, 148, 230–31, 238, 244
Rook, Nina, 102, 107, 225
Rorty, Melitta, 9, 17, 92, 117, 188, 254, 256, 258
Rosen, Richard, 21–23, 196–99, 220
Rosenthal, Elissa, 210

Salamba Adho Mukha Svanasana, 24, 27
Salamba Balasana. *See* Supported Child's pose
Salamba Prasarita Padottanasana. *See* Supported Wide-Legged Standing Forward Bend
Salamba Sarvangasana. *See* Shoulderstand
Salamba Setu Bandhasana. *See* Supported Bridge
Salamba Supta Sukasana. *See* Supported Reclined Crossed Legs
Salamba Urdhva Dhanurasana. *See* Supported Backbend

Salamba Uttanasana. *See* Supported Standing Forward Bend
Salzberg, Sharon, 91, 92, 145, 216, 218, 233
samadhi, 203
samatva. *See* equanimity
Sama Vritti. *See* Equal Ratio Breath
Samkhya, 228
Sanskrit, 210
Satterfield, Jill, 200–201
satya (truthfulness), 140, 169, 237
satyagraha (nonviolent passive resistance), 258
Savasana, 28–35, 62
in bed, 173
contraindications for, 29
as final pose, 161, 185
impermanence in, 226
as meditation, 28–29, 73, 221
pranayama in, 221
Prone, 32, 39, 105, 108, 150, 266
resting in, 161, 266
Restorative, 31
Side-lying, 32
Supported, 30, 39, 81, 125, 152
tips for, 34–35
variations of, 29–33
with chair, 30, 128
Seated Forward Bend, Supported, 58, 95, 107, 114, 150–51
seated yoga poses, 19, 180, 220. *See also* chairs; Easy Sitting pose
self-compassion, 248
self-inquiry, 171, 139, 236–42
self-regulation, 15–16, 89–90
breathing for, 189, 191–94
sense perception, 42–45, 154, 212, 215–16, 244

sense withdrawal, 35

sequences

Active Anger Practice, 98–99

Active Practice for Fear or Anxiety, 111–12

Active Uplifting Practice, 127–28

Afternoon Stress Management Practice, 80–81

Brief Respite Practice, 46–47

Calming Anger Practice, 100–101

Calming Practice for Fear or Anxiety, 113–14

Calming Uplifting Practice, 135–36

Evening Stress Management Practice, 82–84

Fatigue Practice, 158–59

Morning Stress Management Practice, 78–79

Moving Through Grief Practice, 162–63

Releasing Physical Tension, 52–54

Taking a Break from Grief Practice, 165–67

Ser, Shari, 265

Setu Bandhasana. *See* Bridge pose

sexual restraint, 140

shoulder openers, 49, 51, 52, 120, 129

Shoulderstand (Salamba Sarvangasana), 93, 267

alternatives to, 183

Chair, 23

Supported, 26, 27

Shvetashvatara-Upanishad, 190

Side Plank pose, at wall (Vasisthasana), 167, 183

Side-lying Savasana, 32

Sideways Mountain pose, 53

Sikhism, 230

Sirsasana, 93, 183, 267

Skull Shining Breath, 198–200

as stimulating, 191, 193

See also Kapalabhati

sleep

improving (*see* insomnia)

relaxation vs., 28

social justice, 254, 257–59

acceptance and, 224

anger and, 91

grief and, 146

nonviolence and, 139

Somerstein, Lynn, 90, 92, 94, 137

on anxiety, 103, 104, 106

on depression, 115, 117, 118, 122, 131, 133, 205

on grief, 143, 145, 146, 147, 160

Soprasaya, 172

sound, meditating on, 209, 214–15

spirituality, 226–31

Standing Cow-Face pose, 121, 129, 177

Half-, 52, 166

Standing Forward Bend (Uttanasana), 49, 50, 93, 96

as final pose, 161

modifications to, 177, 183

in sequences, 79, 112, 163

Supported (*see* Supported Standing Forward Bend)

at wall, 99, 167

Wide-Legged (*see* Wide-Legged Standing Forward Bend)

Standing Half-Cow Face pose, 52, 166

Standing Leg Stretch (Utthita Hasta Padangusthasana), 180, 183

Standing Locust, 52, 121, 125, 129, 166

standing poses, 89, 180

for anger, 93

for anxiety, 105
for depression, 120, 129
for meditation, 221
as modification, 182–83
modifications of, 176, 177–78, 181–82
stress, 65–84
acute vs. chronic, 67–68
anger and, 87, 90, 97
anxiety and, 109
definition of, 66–67
depression and, 119
emotions and, 68–70, 87–89
grief and, 145, 157
physical symptoms of, 240
practices to manage, 70–77, 191–94
sequences for, 77–84
societal, 2, 67, 116, 143–44
stretching, 48–54
poses for, 52–54
timing of, 50
Sturis, Robin, 153, 154–55
Sukasana. *See* Easy Sitting pose
Sun Salutations (Surya Namaskar), 130, 162,
163, 182
supine poses. *See* reclined poses
Supported Backbend, 39, 53, 127, 136
Supported Bow, 128
Supported Bridge, 24, 25, 27, 132, 161, 183
in sequences, 84, 136
Supported Child's pose, 38, 58, 161
props for, 36, 182
as comforting, 20, 62, 105, 108, 150
in sequences, 81, 152
Supported Downward-Facing Dog, 24, 27
Supported Easy Sitting Forward Bend, 39,
113, 158

supported inversions, 23–27, 62
for anger, 93
for anxiety, 89, 105
blood pressure and, 24–25
contraindications for, 25, 267
for depression, 121, 130
for insomnia, 57
modifications of, 183–84
for stress, 74–75, 82–84
timing of, 25
Supported Legs Up the Wall. *See* Legs
Up the Wall
Supported Locust, 128
Supported Plow, 23, 26, 27
Supported Prone Twist, 39, 81, 152
Supported Reclined Cobbler's pose, 36, 158
Supported Reclined Crossed Legs, 125
Supported Savasana, 30, 39, 81, 125, 152
Supported Seated Forward Bend, 58, 95, 107,
114, 150–51
Supported Shoulderstand, 26, 27
Supported Standing Forward Bend, 24, 26, 27,
93, 96
in sequences, 83, 100, 159
Supported Straight Legs Forward Bend, 114
Supported Wide-Legged Seated Forward
Bend, 114
Supported Wide-Legged Standing Forward
Bend, 27, 93, 183
in sequences, 26, 83, 101, 159
with table, 96
Support pose, 172
Supta Baddha Konasana. *See* Reclined
Cobbler's pose
Supta Bharadvajasana, 20
Supta Padangusthasana, 49, 180

Surya Namaskar, 130, 162, *163*, 182
sympathetic joy (*mudita*), 211, 249–50

tables
    as body support, 179, 181, 183
    as head support, 95, 96, 107
Tadasana. *See* Mountain pose
Tantra Illuminated (Wallis), 187, 213, 233, 234
Tantra yoga, 228–29, 234–36
    ego in, 233
    emotions in, 86
    hatha yoga and, 224
    meditation in, 202, 203, 204, 212, 213
    pranayama in, 191
    on self-inquiry, 237
    sensations in, 41, 212
tarka (discernment), 234–36
tension, releasing physical, 48–54, 160
thoughts
    accepting, 231–34
    emotions and, 69–70
    inquiry into, 236–40, 241–42
    meditation on, 201–2, 204, 217–18
Tigunait, Pandit Rajmani, 248
trataka (gazing), 209
trauma, 212, 232, 252–53
    contraindications for, 205, 239–40
Tree pose (Vrksasana), 47, 177, 178, 181
Triangle pose, 79, 112, 161
    variations of, 174, 177
Trishikhi Brahmana Upanishad, 243
truthfulness, 140, 169, 237. *See also* satya
    (truthfulness)
twists, 20, 97, 175, 178, 268
    Prone, 20, 39, 81, 152
    Reclined, 54, 120, 128, 129
    Seated, 158

Ujjayi pranayama, 191
universal kindness, 140, 211, 244–54
Upanishads, 190, 230, 243
upeksha (equanimity), 211, 250–52
Upward Facing Dog pose, 162
Ustrasana, 178
Uttanasana. *See* Standing Forward Bend
Utthita Hasta Padangusthasana, 180, 183
Utthita Parsvakonasana, 47, 177, *182*

vairagya (nonattachment), 242–44
Vasisthasana, *183*
Vedanta, 227, 228–29
Veterans Yoga Project, 70
Vijnana Bhairava, 213
Viloma pranayama, 193
Viniyoga, 174
vinyasas, 50, 106, 121, 130, 161
    mini, 93, 97, 122–24
violence, 88, 139–40, 203, 236, 251
Virasana, *19*, 219
Vishama Vritti (Extending the Exhalation),
    84, 101, 197
visualization, 209
    for letting go, 243–44
    in postures, 35, 38
    of postures, 173
Vrksasana, 47, 177, *178*, *181*

Wagner, Patrice Priya, 209
Walden, Patricia, 125, 133, 179
Wallis, Christopher, 146, 233, 234, 237
    on being present, 187, 188, 219
    on meditation, 203, 212, 213
Wall Side Plank, *167*, 183
Wall Standing, *54*
Wall Standing Forward Bend, 99, *167*

wall support, 177–78, 182–83, 220

Warrior 1, 45
  modifications of, 176, 177, 178
  in sequences, 98, 135, 167

Warrior 2, 45, 78
  modifications of, 124, 176, 177
  in sequences, 46, 78, 98, 111, 135, 166

Warrior 3, 99, 135
  modifications of, 175, 176, 178

Why Buddhism Is True (Wright), 4, 10, 68,
  200, 241

Wide-Legged Standing Forward Bend, 79,
  112, 183
  Supported (*see* Supported Wide-Legged
  Standing Forward Bend)

Wisdom of Yoga, The (Cope), 245

witnessing, 21, 94, 153–56, 207. *See also*
  meditation; self-inquiry

Wright, Robert, 4, 10, 68, 69, 70, 200, 241

wrist issues, 183

yamas (guiding principles), 12, 139–41, 235–37,
  244–52
  compassion, 141, 211, 247–49, 257
  equanimity, 211, 250–52
  forgiveness, 141, 155, 252–54
  honesty, 171, 236–42
  nonattachment, 242–44
  nonviolence, 139–40, 169, 203, 236, 246
  sympathetic joy, 211, 249–50
  unconditional friendship, 73, 203, 211,
    246–47

yoga
  benefits of, 11–13
  definitions of, 9

history of, 172, 173–74, 190, 224
  philosophy of (*see* yamas; yoga
    philosophy)
  religion and, 231

Yoga as Medicine (McCall), 116

Yoga for Healthy Aging (Zolotow), xiv, 196

Yoga for Healthy Aging Blog, 137, 143, 145, 147,
  148, 153, 156, 160, 236, 237, 241

yoga nidra, 61, 73, 157, 164, 212

Yoga of Breath, The (Rosen), 21, 196

yoga philosophy, 13, 148, 223–59
  action in, 254–59
  attraction and aversion in, 4–6
  change in, 2–4, 8–13, 223–25
  Classical vs. Tantric, 224, 226–29
  eternal in, 226–31
  ethics in (*see* yamas)
  exercises to experience, 226, 229, 234
  ego in, 233–34
  letting go in, 234–54
  nonattachment in, 242–44
  self-inquiry in, 234–42

Yoga Sutras (Patanjali), 224
  on afflictions, 5, 6
  alternative systems to, 224, 255
  Bryant on, 10, 172
  on cultivating the opposite, 244–45
  on dualism, 227–28, 233
  eightfold path in, 75–76, 190, 203
  on equanimity, 250–51
  on friendship, 246
  on meditation, 203, 204
  on pranayama, 189–90
  yamas in, 140, 235, 237, 251, 255

Yoga Yajnavalkya, 171, 236, 253